Sin in the City

By the Same Authors

Girls in Trouble: Sexuality and Social Control in Rural Scotland, 1660–1780
Rosalind Mitchison and Leah Leneman
1 898218 89 7

Sin in the City

Sexuality and Social
Control in Urban Scotland
1660–1780

Leah Leneman and Rosalind Mitchison

SCOTTISH CULTURAL PRESS
EDINBURGH

First published in 1998 by
Scottish Cultural Press
Unit 14, Leith Walk Business Centre
130 Leith Walk, Edinburgh EH6 5DT
Tel: 0131 555 5950 • Fax: 0131 555 5018
e-mail: scp@sol.co.uk

Copyright © Leah Leneman and Rosalind Mitchison 1998

All rights reserved. No part of the publication may be reproduced, stored in a retrieval system, or transmitted in any form or by any means, electronic, digital, mechanical, photocopying, recording or otherwise, without prior permission of Scottish Cultural Press

British Library Cataloguing in Publication Data
A catalogue record for this book is available from the British Library

ISBN: 1 898218 90 0

Printed and bound by
Interprint Ltd, Malta

Contents

List of Figures		vi
List of Tables		vi
Acknowledgements		vii
	Introduction	1
1	Setting the Scene	4
2	The Mechanisms of Social Control	19
3	Control of Non-Sexual Offences	40
4	The Background to Illegitimacy and Bridal Pregnancy	50
	Appendix 1: Bond signed by midwives, Edinburgh St Cuthbert's	67
5	Illegitimacy and Bridal Pregnancy	69
	Appendix 2: List of kirk session registers used	81
6	Evading and Defying Discipline	82
7	Lying to the Session	98
	Appendix 3: Case History 1 – Aberdeen	116
	Appendix 4: Case History 2 – Edinburgh St Cuthbert's	118
	Appendix 5: Case History 3 – Aberdeen	120
	Appendix 6: Case History 4 – South Leith	122
	Appendix 7: Case History 5 – Edinburgh St Cuthbert's	124
	Appendix 8: Case History 6 – Glasgow Govan	126
8	The Rise and Rise of Irregular Marriage	128
	Appendix 9: Total irregular marriages in parishes with long runs	145
	Appendix 10: Marriage Case History 1 – South Leith	146
	Appendix 11: Marriage Case History 2 – South Leith	148
	Appendix 12: Marriage Case History 3 – Edinburgh Canongate	150
	Appendix 13: Marriage Case History 4 – Edinburgh Trinity College	152
	Appendix 14: Marriage Case History 5 – Glasgow Govan	154
	Appendix 15: Marriage Case History 5 – Dundee	156
	Conclusion	159
	Index	161

List of Figures

5.1	Illegitimacy ratios: South Leith and Aberdeen	73
5.2	Illegitimacy ratios: Trinity College and Old Aberdeen	73
5.3	Illegitimacy ratios: Dundee	74
5.4	Illegitimacy ratios: Govan, Barony and St Cuthbert's	76

List of Tables

4.1	Months pregnant when discovered by session: South Leith	52
4.2	Months pregnant when discovered by session: Aberdeen St Nicholas	52
4.3	Months pregnant when discovered by session: Dundee	53
5.1	Admission percentages	74
5.2	Percentage of total cases which involved repeaters	78
8.1	Numbers cited at different periods of time after an irregular marriage: Edinburgh St Cuthbert's	140
8.2	Numbers cited at different periods of time after an irregular marriage: North Leith	140
8.3	Numbers cited at different periods of time after an irregular marriage: South Leith	140

Acknowledgements

We are very grateful to the ESRC for funding the first phase of our research, and to the Leverhulme Trust for funding the second phase. Without their financial assistance this book could not have been written.

The staff of the Scottish Record Office, Strathclyde Regional Archive, Dundee City Archive, Aberdeen City Archive, and Edinburgh City Archive were unfailingly helpful in every way.

Over many years our research has been underpinned by the encouragement and hospitality of the Department of Economic and Social History, University of Edinburgh.

The work of scholars on the Scottish cities in the seventeenth and eighteenth centuries has enabled us to place our own findings in context; their writings are cited in the footnotes to Chapter 1.

Introduction

Sexual activity is an important part of human life, yet only recently has it received close attention from serious historians. This is surprising considering its multifaceted significance. It has been the self-expression of individuals, the source of a large body of poetry, the basis of the arrangements for the transfer of property between different generations and is a vital component in population growth or decline. A sign of its importance is the effort made by many different societies to regulate it, and in particular to confine it within marriage. The regulation of marriage is also a mixture of expressed rules and of silent but assumed conventions.

We have already produced one study based on the investigations of the Church of Scotland into sexual activity outwith the accepted systems of marriage. This made use of the records of discipline in the Church's archives of seventy-eight rural and small town parishes and was published in 1989 as *Sexuality and Social Control: Scotland 1660–1780*. The Church of Scotland maintained an active and effective system of investigation and discipline of social offences long after anything of this type had been abandoned by other state churches, and its records are readily available. The original impetus of our earlier work had been an attempt to quantify illegitimacy and to see if in the early-modern period this had the same striking regional pattern which it had in mid-Victorian Scotland. Because we did not think that the Church would have been able to carry out its investigations into sexual behaviour effectively in the cities we did not include these in our sample.[1]

Our work on that earlier book widened our field of interest because our sources did much more than simply record and penalise the production of illegitimate children. We were able to expand our concern with illegitimacy into a more general concern with sexual nonconformity as the Church perceived it.[2] Also, the attitudes and actions of individuals who came before the church courts – individuals mainly of humble means whose lives are not otherwise documented in the historical record – were brought to life, often in their own words, by conscientious clerks. But what also became clear was that the ministers and the kirk sessions (the courts that operated at parish level) could effectively trace sinners who had run away to the city to avoid the discipline system of rural parishes. In spite of the relative anonymity of the city scene, ministers who wrote to enquire about men or women believed to have gone to a city were often answered with precise information. It appeared that the system was functioning not only in smaller settlements but in urban areas as well. So we planned a further research project.

There has been considerable historical interest in illegitimacy over the last twenty years. This is partly because it is a component in basic demographic features. Illegitimacy levels vary markedly and between different countries and with interesting trends over time.[3] The case of Scotland has particular interest because from the mid-nineteenth century it had two regions which persistently showed remarkably high levels well into the twentieth century.[4] For the earlier period which we studied these were not yet established, but there were still interesting regional differences then and trends in some areas were marked. It was obvious that we needed to study the urban scene.

Urban history is a subject of increasing attention and during the last twenty years has become recognised as a specific area of research. For Scotland most of the work had until recently been concerned with developments since 1800, but there have recently been important studies for earlier periods.[5] The study of Scotland, a country with its own law and church system, gives opportunities for perceiving the effects of the sudden urban growth of the later eighteenth century, as well as the gradual effect of English influence as the two countries grew nearer to each other. For us a valuable separate feature is the distinct record system produced by the country's Church courts, a source not available at the same period for England. The Calvinist dogma of the Scottish Church led to the maintenance of a system of parish discipline not to be found in the eighteenth-century Anglican Church except for a while in the Isle of Man. Anglican Church discipline in any case had never been very effective, for secular lawyers had been able to do much to frustrate it, and its greater formality imposed costs on people which they could not meet.[6] It did not survive into the later seventeenth century, whereas the Scottish system worked until the late eighteenth century.

The difference in the temporal span of these systems means that it is possible in the Scottish material to see what happens when the relatively backward and stagnant economy of Scotland moved suddenly into the pre-industrial growth of the later eighteenth century. The Scottish cities were transformed by this surge in growth, and in other ways by significant cultural developments. So the urban scene in Scotland in our period has particular interest. Economic and cultural change were very rapid developments.

The research for this book has shown us that sexual issues involved considerable interaction between different social groups. Upper-class men frequently looked for sexual satisfaction among the lower classes. All levels of society appear to have been remarkably articulate, and ready to express themselves on the nature of marriage. In particular many couples had their own idea of what was a valid marriage and how it should be established. In the later eighteenth century two of our parishes in particular, covering the suburban areas of Glasgow and Edinburgh, had session clerks with the interests of social anthropologists. These men reported what was said by offenders and witnesses with remarkable fullness. We are therefore able to set out in extraordinary detail the views of many types of people on the nature of marriage and other sexual relationships, and of their responses to authority. Social control was by then slipping from the Church, but it had survived long enough to give us an intimate view of the opinions and actions of a wide range of people.

Even today the cities of Scotland display very different features. They did so also in our period of research. It is our regret that the records surviving are not more complete, but even so the richness which we have found is one of the rewards of research, and can be shared by readers of this book.

Notes

1 The starting and closing dates chosen for this and our earlier research were determined by a desire to keep clear of the disturbances of the revolutionary period in the mid-seventeenth century, and by the evident decline in the whole system of discipline by the Church of Scotland in the 1780s.
2 The Church required firm evidence for cases brought to its court system, and had a relatively narrow concept of proof: the production of a child out of wedlock or within nine months of marriage was evidence of unmarried sexual intercourse, and so was the evidence of witnesses to intercourse, but nothing else. As a result the Church courts provide us with no information on homosexual practices, paedophilia, or intercourse with girls too young for conception. Since most children left their parental home in their early teens to work and live in the home of another family our research has produced no information on incest within the immediate family.
3 Peter Laslett, Karla Oosterveen and Richard M. Smith (eds.), *Bastardy and its Comparative History* (London, 1980). Richard Adair, 'Two Englands? Regional variation in Bastardy and Courtship 1538–1700', in R.M. Smith (ed.), *Regional and Spatial Demographic Patterns in the Past* (forthcoming).
4 T.C. Smout, 'Aspects of Sexual Behaviour in Nineteenth-Century Scotland', in Laslett, Oosterveen and Smith, *Bastardy*, pp. 192–216. Andrew Blaikie, *Illegitimacy, Sex and Society: Northern Scotland 1750–1900* (Oxford, 1993).
5 Michael Lynch (ed.), *The Early Modern Town in Scotland* (London, 1983).
6 E.H. Stenning, 'Manx Spiritual Laws', *Isle of Man History and Antiquarian Society Proceedings V* (1942–50), pp. 287–97. Martin Ingram, *Church Courts, Sex and Marriage in England 1570–1640* (Cambridge, 1987).

1

Setting the Scene

In 1660 Scotland was a poor and relatively undeveloped country, but it was unmistakably part of western Christendom. All European governments then held that it was desirable that a state should be unified in religious allegiance. For the most part Scotland had accepted Calvinism in the Reformation period and had, over the following century, set up an effective preaching ministry in the lowland areas and achieved a general adherence to Calvinism by the population. Catholicism continued in parts of the north-east and in the highlands: the Catholic mass was formally illegal but it survived where the nobility still favoured it and in remote areas. For most of Scotland the dominant social features of Calvinism were well established: regular attendance in a bare church on Sundays to hear long sermons, little ceremonial for rites of passage, impromptu prayers of great length, catechising of the household by the minister, annual communions for those accepted as worthy. In all aspects of religious life the absence of pageantry and ceremony had become a ceremony of its own. Government of the parish in religious and moral matters was by the kirk session, made up of the minister and elders, all men, of course.

Calvinist teaching, as accepted in Scotland, laid down that a godly discipline was one of the signs of a true Church, and membership of a true Church was necessary if men were to know that they were predestined for salvation. Godly discipline was thus an essential part of life. To enforce it the Church of Scotland had erected a structure of courts. The lowest of these, with the greatest impact on the community, was the kirk session: above that came the presbytery, where the centre of church power was supposed to lie. There were two higher courts, the synod and the General Assembly: these met twice and once a year respectively. The presbytery met every few weeks, and the attendance of parish ministers was compulsory. The kirk session met as parish business required, usually on Sunday after sermon. Its field of action was parish business, the sustenance of the poor and discipline.

Because discipline was embodied in a court, it concentrated on offences which could be legally proved. This meant that many sins were ignored. No attention was paid to spiritual pride, avaricious behaviour, selfishness or greed unless these sins led to actions which were reported by witnesses and regarded as unchristian. What was prosecuted by the session was failure to observe the Sabbath, excessive brutality within the family, quarrelling or fighting with neighbours, conspicuous drunkenness, swearing in public, failure to attend church and extra-marital sexual behaviour either directly observed or resulting in the pregnancy of an unmarried woman. The sessions investigating these matters appear not to have considered other sexual irregularities, such as paedophilia or homosexuality, though any overt physical intimacy such as holding hands or embracing would also be censured under the general title of 'scandalous carriage'.

On sexual matters the Church held that intercourse should be confined to married

1: Setting the Scene

couples. Monogamous marriage was available to all adults except those barred by nearness of kin or affinity. The Church defined as adult a boy of fourteen and a girl of twelve, but in practice marriage was usually much later. It was taken for granted that a married couple meant a separate household, and a reasonable prospect of economic self-sufficiency. This did not usually happen until the couple were in their later twenties. Servants and apprentices, living in their masters' houses, were not free to marry. Many people never attained the economic independence considered suitable for marriage.

Marriage was supposed to be monogamous and permanent, but divorce was accepted by both Church and state, for adultery or for desertion. All sexual activity outside marriage was labelled by the Church as fornication, or if one party was married, adultery. The latter was a very serious offence. If an unmarried woman gave birth, fornication was regarded as proved. If a child was born to a married couple less than nine calendar months after marriage, that too was evidence of fornication: 'antenuptial uncleanness' it was called, and was ground for Church prosecution.

The pattern of relatively late marriage meant that there was a large number of sexually mature adults not free to marry. The cramped nature of most of the houses in which they lived gave them physical closeness to servants of the other sex. Many households occupied only one or two rooms. Furniture and space were sparse. People shared beds, usually three at a time, though the Church on various occasions objected to mixed sexes in the same bed. Altogether material circumstances put a considerable strain on chastity, but the Church made no allowance for this.

Scotland's adherence to European norms is shown in her town structure. Towns were privileged and chartered societies, given certain rights of self-government in return for certain payments, either to King or noble. They contained merchants and craftsmen, as well as unprivileged labourers. Rural society came to towns to buy metal goods, tools, and leather goods and to sell farm produce, textiles etc. The knitting of stockings, spinning and weaving of low grade linen or woollen cloth, were all rural activities. Much of this was for home use, but if it was for sale it would be brought to a town.

The family was supposed to be separately housed; family here means the kin group and their servants. But this did not always happen. Housing materials were expensive and building took time. A big fire in 1624 in Dunfermline is evidence of this: it left homeless 287 families by the destruction of 220 houses.[1] Much urban housing was what we would call flats. The householder was master of the family. He was supposed to control and rule wife, children and servants, and this control included the right, indeed the duty, to beat them, so long as such beating did not cause permanent damage or loud outcry, and did not take place on Sunday. Women and children over some young age (eight was normal) were expected to be contributing to the household's earnings or support, unless the children were at school. Children were expected to have joined the Christian community by baptism as infants, and by around eight to understand religious doctrine. They would be catechised each year by the minister. Between ten and fifteen many children left home to enter service, to become either servant or apprentice in the household of another family, and to be under the discipline of other adults. The norms of family life were authoritarian, yet the existence in burghs of ale houses meant that there were places and occasions of relaxation and opportunities for young people to get together.

The Scottish cities examined here are Edinburgh (and its satellites, Canongate and Leith), Glasgow, Dundee and Aberdeen and we have studied them for the period 1660–1780. At the start of this period only Edinburgh was truly a city, with the population, functions, institutions and economic links appropriate to the status; the others were still just large towns which might or might not develop into cities. (Indeed another large town, Perth, which we have not included in this study, was in 1660 of a similar size and economic strength to Aberdeen but did not in our period make the transition.) Urban growth in Scotland was very slow at first but came with a rush after 1750, when in a few decades Scotland passed from being one of the least urbanised states in Europe to being one of the most urban.[2]

Towns were not communities of equals; they contained a wide range of wealth and income. There were two important divisions within all urban communities, between merchants and craftsmen and between free – the burgesses – and unfree. The word merchant covers a wide range of wealth and activity, from a trader in foreign goods, often owning a share in a ship, maintaining his affairs by a skilful use of credit, to a packman or chapman walking the roads and carrying his capital stock on his back. In all urban constitutions, town setts they were called, the merchants dominated the council. Free merchants belonged to the merchant guild, free craftsmen to the craft incorporations which provided a lesser share of the council. But some craftsmen might be in the merchant guild, and some merchants might have the freedom of another burgh. The rigidities of the definitions were succumbing to the powerful influence of economic change.[3]

The large towns also contained people of standing, gentry and professional people. The gentry, mostly nearby landowners, might be temporary visitors or have a permanent home in the town. Their specialised needs would have an important influence on the trade and occupations of the city. In particular it was they who demanded professional services, from lawyers, doctors, surgeons and apothecaries and teachers, as well as encouraging the luxury crafts and trades: hair and wig dressers, milliners and mantua makers, booksellers and printers, wine merchants and coffee houses. Lawyers were necessary for will making, for marriage settlements, for all transfers of land, and for the conduct and resolution of quarrels with neighbouring landowners. Physicians were the source of diagnosis and advice about health and disease, surgeons were useful for bleeding and other approved remedies, apothecaries for drugs and advice, for purgatives, poultices and plasters. In Edinburgh the incorporation of surgeon apothecaries always provided a member of the town council. Gentry used the large towns for education for their children; schools, dancing and fencing masters were needed. Gentry might come to town for an important wedding or to have a son and heir baptised. The large towns were also, in the later seventeenth century beginning to provide recreational facilities for the upper classes.

Towns were very different places from their rural hinterlands, but there was constant interaction between the two societies. Towns still had a share in farming; their own harvest called for labour from the urban community. Cattle were walked to town for slaughter, and other goods were brought in to the markets. Coal was shipped from the collieries near the sea or came into town in carts. Landowners in the mid-seventeenth century still received the bulk of their rents in grain although they were keen to increase the role of money, and had to organise transport and sale. In times of harvest failure the rural labour force flocked to towns hoping for work, or

1: Setting the Scene

at least to be in a place where there might be grain imports.

Inevitably the ability of the Church to impose discipline, especially sexual discipline, was less accepted, and less enforceable, in a large town than in the country. As the towns expanded it became difficult to keep their entire population under surveillance. All these towns were ports, or in the case of Edinburgh, controlled an adjacent port, Leith. They were Royal Burghs, which meant that they shared the privilege of foreign trade, in return for carrying a burden of taxation. The goods that came in from abroad went on to the rural hinterland, from which much of the exports came. The industries of the towns, small scale though they were, created a demand for labour which was supplied by the adolescents and young adults of the hinterland. There was also a demand for domestic servants, particularly for women. So the towns had many links with the countryside, and contained large populations of young single adults, particularly women in insecure and vulnerable positions.

Our study of rural Scotland started out as an exploration of illegitimacy in the different regions and over time, and then expanded into the whole subject of social control. Similarly, this project began as a comparison of illegitimacy ratios in Scottish cities where such figures could be elicited, and it was our discovery of how different from rural Scotland the situation was in those cities that made us go on to a full scale investigation of 'sin' and social control in urban Scotland. The collection of illegitimacy figures from kirk session registers still formed the core of the project, but the wealth of qualitative material found provided scope for an attempt to understand how control was enforced – and resisted – in this urban environment.

In justifying our original study we commented that illegitimacy is of importance because it is an indicator of rule breaking, its existence being proof that the generally accepted Christian principle which confined sexual activity to marriage had been disregarded. Also, historians have used illegitimacy study as a route to understanding the views and feelings of the common people, especially of women. As will be made clear in a later chapter, measuring illegitimacy proved far more difficult for cities than for rural areas, but session clerks in cities recorded in far more depth and detail aspects of behaviour and discipline, providing many insights into the mental world of those who broke the rules.

Social control begins with the family. At that level it is not measurable, but parents accept (or do not accept) a set of social mores from above. Our study is based on those imposed by the ecclesiastical courts. Unlike England, and most other western European countries, social control by the church in Scotland went on into the late eighteenth century. Naturally, social control by civil authorities was also omnipresent, and in our next chapter we explore the relationship between those two authorities in our cities, but whereas for the most part only law breakers came into contact with magistrates, nearly everyone went to church and was there indoctrinated with certain principles and moral values.

The late seventeenth century was a period of sharp change in the urban pattern. Many new towns were founded; a town could not come into existence without a charter, the grant of market rights and a sett, but many of these new foundations, and some older ones, never developed a real economic role. Middling sized towns in many parts of Europe were in decline. Our big four – Edinburgh, Aberdeen, Glasgow and Dundee – were, however, gradually separating themselves from the rest of the Royal Burghs. Already they paid nearly two thirds of the tax on the Royal Burghs.

Scotland has always been a country of marked regional differences, so it is no surprise that her cities have had, and still have, distinctive personalities. Aberdeen was the most conspicuously dedicated to trade.[4] Merchants dominated numerically, by 250 to 350 among the burgesses, yet her trade was not doing well. It had been largely based on the export of coarse woollens, and the demand for these was drying up. She had had a bad time in the period of revolution and war, since the attachment of the north-east to episcopacy had brought down covenanting wrath. Thomas Tucker, sent by Cromwell to inspect the ports of Scotland in 1656, said that she was 'noe despicable burgh'.[5] Before the Great Rebellion her population had lain between 8,000 and 9,000: now in 1660 this was down to about 7,500. An English regiment had been quartered on the town for much of the 1650s, which in economic effect could be seen as the equivalent of a tourist industry, but now that had gone, and even its adjacent burgh, Old Aberdeen was trying to enter into rivalry with it.

We have included Old Aberdeen in our study because, though only a small place, it had features appropriate to a city, an episcopal see and a university, King's College, a rival to Marischal College in Aberdeen and described by Tucker as 'the cheife Academie of Scotland'. Old Aberdeen had had a population of about 1,500, but this had risen to 1,800, perhaps even higher. By the time of the hearth tax of 1691 she had a surprisingly large number of 'paid hearths', but this figure is difficult to interpret in terms of population in a town containing an unusually large number of big houses. Her increase seems to have been due to a policy of rivalry with Aberdeen over markets. Eighteen hundred or even 2,000 by the end of the century appears to have been the peak population produced by this policy.[6]

Aberdeen's outside province was distinctively her own, and strengthened by the existence of the Universities. Landed gentry would find it a long journey to use the facilities of Edinburgh, though sooner of later most of them would do so. but the poll tax records for 1696 do not show many professional men in the two towns; the ministers, of course, some regents at the Universities, ten lawyers and seven medical men.[7]

Aberdeen paid 5 per cent of the tax on the Royal Burghs: Dundee paid 4 per cent. But earlier in the century Dundee's share had been 11 per cent. The change is a measure of what she had suffered in the wars. Tucker's account of Dundee was not particularly sympathetic, for he was an Englishman: 'sometime a towne of riches and trade... her obstinacy and pride of late yeares rendring her a prey to soldiers'; but he added 'though not glorious, yett not contemptible'. The 'obstinacy' had meant the sack of 1651 in which 2,000 are thought to have perished. The later seventeenth century was a bad time for all the Tay ports. Leith monopolised much of the east coast export trade, the markets for low quality cloth were contracting and the series of wars with the Netherlands made north sea trade risky. It was linen which rescued Dundee, but this industry and trade did not become significant until the 1740s. Dundee had troubles about sandbanks in the Tay estuary and her harbour's exposure to wind. In the 1660s her population was probably a little over 8,000; in the hearth tax of 1691 she had 100 more paying hearths than Aberdeen, suggesting nearly 500 more people. Her recovery from the war period had been slow for her business was with everyday useful commodities which had a relatively static demand, linen cloth and thread, leather, soap, rope, to which she later added glass and sugar. She brought in flour and flax from the Baltic and everyday necessities such as tools from the Netherlands. Her province, Angus, Kinross-shire and Fife, was not immune to poaching by either Aberdeen or Edinburgh, particularly the latter which could offer

1: Setting the Scene

more sophisticated amenities.[8]

The seventeenth century had seen some difficult times for Glasgow. She experienced two devastating fires (in 1652 and 1677) which led to a greater use of stone in building. She was much involved in the covenanting resistance to the policy of the restored monarchy, leading to fines and the quartering of soldiers. Her share in the Revolution of 1688–9 in troops and money left her on the edge of bankruptcy.[9]

Nevertheless, the period as a whole was more conspicuous for the city's achievements. She had been gaining in economic and political terms and in 1670 she was acknowledged as second in the ranks of Royal Burghs, with a tax share of 20 per cent, when Edinburgh paid 37 per cent. At the start of the century she had stood fifth. Her nineteenth century demographer, James Cleland, estimated her population in 1660 as 14,700,[10] but more recent estimates would lower this. It is not the actual level of population which is striking but the fact that it certainly rose during the seventeenth century by at least a half. In its own buoyant manner Glasgow was moving into the small group of large towns in Britain which besides the great town of London contained Bristol and Norwich. She carried a fair sized group of craftsmen, to whom she gave a greater share in representation on the council than did most Royal Burghs, but her growth was based on trade; with the west coast ports of England, with Ulster and with the English colonies, which last, by the English Navigation Acts, should before the 1707 Act of Union have been confined to English ships and English ports. In the seventeenth century her trade with Argyll and the Western Isles was of great importance. She also traded with Ireland. After 1707 her overland trade with England developed, and was particularly important in enabling her to stock her stores in America. With the encouragement of the Privy Council she was experimenting in the 1680s with new industries. She had a university and an archiepiscopal see. Her long term problem was the navigation of the Clyde: the river was dredged in the later eighteenth century to make a narrow channel usable but not till the nineteenth century could big ships get up it. But the city overcame this handicap by developing Port Glasgow as her outlet. She also used the land link to Bo'ness for trade with France and the Netherlands. Craftsmen were important to the city for she offered the services of their skills to a large region. Her herring curing, for instance, gave an outlet for fishing to the ports of Argyll and Ayrshire, and food to many.[11]

Edinburgh has to be seen as a complex structure. In population she was the second city of Britain. Recent estimates give her, with her satellites, over 40,000 in the 1690s, a figure based on 14,343 tax paying hearths.[12] She had rather less in 1660, for the 1690s figure was almost certainly enhanced by having for a time housed a royal court, that of James VII, then Duke of York, when exiled from England to avoid provoking the Exclusionist party.[13] All sorts of sophisticated crafts and activities could be promoted by a court, particularly conspicuous display. The 1694 poll tax shows aspects of this. The city then had 29 wigmakers (wigs were a recent fashion), and, even more significant, these had 39 apprentices, showing the expectation of increasing business. There were over 200 lawyers of one kind or another. The presence of the Court of Session provided many opportunities for lawyers, but their number is also a sign of the presence of gentry from a wide area. There were also 33 physicians, more than the men much more practically useful, the 23 surgeons. Lawyers and physicians were noticeably concentrated in the central parishes of the city.[14]

Sin in the City

Though cities were closely packed communities without socially select areas, there were differences in the dominant occupations of residents in the various parishes of Edinburgh, as shown in the poll tax of 1694. The central parish of the New Kirk, lying to the north of the High Street, contained a third of the city's advocates and 40 per cent of the Writers to the Signet, the two prestigious types of lawyer, 15 per cent of the city's merchants, 18 per cent of the physicians, and 7 per cent of the gentry. It had few craftsmen in the less wealthy activities, only 15 out of 311 tailors, one out of 156 cordiners, and no weavers, candlemakers or cobblers. The other parish in the heart of the city, Old Kirk, lying to the south of the High Street, had fewer gentry: a quarter of its householders were professional men and another quarter craftsmen. Not surprisingly, it had a large number of apprentices and servants, more female servants than any other parish.

Another central parish, Tron, south east of the High Street, had nearly 30 per cent of its households craftsmen, more than any other parish except Canongate, and was also well equipped with professionals. Tolbooth, to the north west, stretching to the Nor' Loch, had almost as high a concentration of merchants as the New Kirk. Lady Yester parish, south of the Tron, contained many of the poorer households; over half of its households had no servants and there were few apprentices, and few children of taxable age. It seems to have been a reservoir of labour. But even in this proletarian area there was a writer, a scatter of brewers and a moderate number of gentry. In Greyfriars parish, the south west, stretching to the West Port, nearly a quarter of the houses were those of merchants, a third were of craftsmen and the range of crafts was wide. Not many gentry lived there but a lot of men working in the luxury trades, for instance there were three wigmakers, a glover and a musician.

Trinity College parish, in the north east of the city, is of particular interest because it has supplied better records than the others. Like all parishes, its population was mixed. It was relatively low in merchants: only 13 per cent of its households were so labelled. Nearly half the houses were of craftsmen, and these included luxury trades, a perfumer, an embroiderer, a silk weaver, a confectioner, two glovers and numerous saddlers.

The West Kirk, or St Cuthbert's, was not yet part of Edinburgh. It wrapped round the city outside the gates. Its pattern of occupations shows its continuing rural character. All the men in Edinburgh classified as tenants lived there, as well as 435 cottars; only one lawyer (an advocate), one surgeon but 55 weavers. It had very few children old enough to be taxed, about one to every four households, whereas in the New Kirk there were five to every four households. It had few apprentices, but a good quantity of male and female servants and nearly a quarter of the city's gentry.[15]

The satellite town of Canongate had some 2,000 poll tax payers, suggesting nearly 5,000 inhabitants. Like Edinburgh she was cramped into a narrow site, and could not easily grow except upwards. She was a craftsmen's town, though there were some large houses in which the aristocracy came to stay for periods. Upward growth meant that social stratification was shown by verticality. The poorer part of society occupied attics or cellars in the large blocks of apartments. Canongate had at one time been Holyrood Abbey's burgh and in the seventeenth century serviced the court centred on the palace of Holyrood. It retained its own character. Nearly 50 per cent of its households were those of craftsmen, and as a result it had few gentry and professional men. It was well supplied with the poorer crafts, particularly with cordiners, but it also had two jewellers and more gunsmiths than any other parish.

1: Setting the Scene

Over half the houses did not have a servant and over a third did not have a taxable child, suggesting that many adolescents had gone to service.[16]

The satellite town of Leith had two parishes, South and North Leith. North Leith was where ships were built, South where they were loaded and unloaded with goods which belonged to the rich merchants in Edinburgh. Both sides had petty craftsmen, mostly poor, and greatly outnumbered by labourers. Together they had a population of between four and five thousand, with somewhat more than two thirds of this in South Leith. That the population of these parishes lacked social distinction is shown by the presence, in South Leith, of a solitary lawyer, no doctors of any kind and none of the more expensive crafts, such as goldsmithing. If seventeenth-century Edinburgh was a merchant's city then Leith was a seaman's town. Skippers were the aristocracy of the seaport.[17]

Both the Leith parishes were markedly more proletarian than those of Edinburgh proper. North Leith had no gentry and very few professional men and merchants. Over 60 per cent of its householders were classified as 'indweller', presumably an available labour force. South Leith, roughly similar, had a few gentry and about a third of its houses were for craftsmen. Apprentices were rare in both parishes. That South Leith still had a rural dimension is shown by the presence of 37 cottars. North Leith's domestic poverty is suggested by the presence there of only 50 female servants, but it was smaller in population than the other parishes, which may explain part of this low level. All the other Edinburgh parishes had over 100 and Old Kirk had over 500.

These figures come from the poll tax, and we do not know the level of poll tax evasion. In an earlier tax schedule nearly a quarter of the city's households were classified as poor. This suggests a life of hardship for the family. The contrast in living standards for these people and the comfortably off gentry and professionals would be sharp.

A city such as Edinburgh (to a lesser degree all these towns) had a population divided by the issue of permanence. On one side was a tight intermarried group of families involved in craft work or trade, the elite of these burgesses carrying on the town's government, presiding over courts or attending the kirk session, and knowing almost everyone in the town. Towns did not have police forces, but some of the citizens had to serve as constables, not a full time occupation, and make sure that the town's regulations, such as those about clearing up after market, were observed. A large town would have the powers of criminal jurisdiction and a prison in which to incarcerate suspects. In a town of less than 10,000 there was little anonymity for anyone. There was also a temporary population, mostly servants. In 1691 Edinburgh had 3,276 female servants and over a thousand men servants, as well as 700 apprentices. Without these people her industries would have been crippled, and the domestic life of many families much more uncomfortable. The demand for female house servants was so great that it distorted the sex ratio of young adults; in the age range of 15 to 24 in Edinburgh there were only 76 males for every hundred females. Some of these incomers would become part of the permanent population of the city; that was the expectation certainly of the apprentices. Others might move back to the country or move to another town.

There was also the temporary population of the landed families which used the facilities of the town, and also visiting merchants and seamen. The richer end of this population was of great importance to the urban economy. It encouraged the luxury trades. It was because the local gentry had relatively low incomes that Dundee's manufactures and trade were in basic rather than in luxury commodities. There were, of course, overlapping areas of demand: Dundee's burgesses consumed large quantities of French and Spanish wine, and to landowners deep drinking was an important activity.

By the mid-seventeenth century all these large towns had recognised that they could not manage on the mediaeval system of a single parish with a single minister. Dundee had three parishes with their own ministers, but these met together in a general session for the whole town. Late in the eighteenth century she added a fourth charge. Aberdeen, though only a single parish, had three ministers, and Old Aberdeen had two. Edinburgh was divided into nine parishes, of which seven covered the central city, though it did not yet have separate churches for all of them. These parishes had their own kirk sessions, but were joined together financially under the town council, which paid the ministers' salaries and controlled spending by the official, the kirk treasurer. Canongate had a single parish with two ministers, so had South Leith; North Leith had a single minister. Glasgow's cathedral church of St Mungo was divided into four charges under the control of the city council, and she also had a further independent charge. Both Edinburgh and Glasgow were wrapped round by a suburban parish, for Edinburgh St Cuthbert's or the West Kirk, for Glasgow Barony: in the seventeenth century these were still rural in their economy, but in the course of the eighteenth century suddenly became fully urbanised. Glasgow still adjoined a mainly rural parish, Govan. It is our regret that only a limited amount of parish material appears to have survived for the kirk sessions of Edinburgh city and none for Glasgow city.

Restoration burgh life was not prosperous except in Edinburgh, where the Scottish Parliament, the Court of Session and the General Assembly of the Church provided business. The much lower level of official business elsewhere is shown by the fact that Aberdeen had, in the poll tax, only eleven lawyers.[18] The end of Cromwell's incorporation into England freed Scottish trade from control by the English Parliament but did not protect Scotland from the effects of the second and third Dutch wars. The aristocracy was heavily burdened by debts incurred during the wars. Grain prices stood low, benefiting the common people, but not landowners. Exports to England of coal and cattle expanded, but neither of these gave business to the cities. Aberdeen and Dundee appear to have had no population growth in the later seventeenth century.

The Revolution of 1689, the change from the rule of the Roman Catholic James VII to the Protestant William and Mary, involved no loss of life in the towns. It was followed by the change from episcopal church government to presbyterian, and this meant that most parish ministers were forced out of their posts. In South Leith and Aberdeen the episcopal ministers held on and for some time there were rival kirk sessions carrying on parish business, including discipline. The city most affected by the change in church government was Edinburgh where many 'outed' ministers collected looking for employment. In the 1694 poll tax Edinburgh, whose parishes held 15 ministers, had 82 ministers and two bishops. The extra men were looking for work as teachers, secretaries, chaplains to noblemen, or ministers to the new dissenting group, the episcopalian conventicles. Many of these were Jacobite by conviction, so though there was as yet no doctrinal difference between the

1: Setting the Scene

established Church and the episcopal Church there was mutual hostility. Many people still preferred baptisms and marriages to be conducted by the episcopal clergy, which meant not only a demarcation dispute over fees but also a breach in the mechanism of church discipline.

The Revolution was accompanied by a new foreign war and a civil war, not circumstances beneficial to urban prosperity. Business men and landowners then also lost considerable sums in the failed Darien scheme of the 1690s. Then the country entered on its last and best remembered general famine, the Ill Years of King William's reign. The harvest was poor in 1695, blighted badly in 1696, 1698, and 1699. Famine-based epidemics swept across the country. Rural society, needing all its resources for food, had no demand for urban products. Farmers refused to take on servants since they could not afford to feed them. Starving country dwellers walked to the nearest towns hoping for work and to be near imported food. The towns could not keep all of them out. We do not know the level of deaths in this disaster, but it was probably over a tenth of the country's population. The famine was particularly severe in Aberdeen.

The eighteenth century was more prosperous than the seventeenth, and the urban communities were abandoning the old, rigid definitions. The royal burghs had lost their monopoly of foreign trade in 1672 but still predominated in it. The barriers between free and unfree and between merchant and craftsmen were being broken or overridden because they no longer fitted the structure of activities. Burgess status in the early eighteenth century became of significance socially and politically but did not define the way in which a living could be earned and opportunities seized. Apprenticeship was still the way to craftsman status, but the length of time required came down then to three years from seven. Merchant houses with foreign links might prefer to send their youths abroad to learn trade in some foreign house. Merchants might have links and burgess status in nearby lesser towns. The various processes of liberalisation were conspicuous in Glasgow but occurred in all the big towns.[19]

The patterns of trade and the functions of towns changed after the 1707 Act of Union with England. It was now legal to trade with the English colonies, but some other trades experienced higher duties. Glasgow in particular benefited both in trade and industry. Repopulation after the famine was quick in all the big towns except Aberdeen, which had been particularly hard hit. In the 1720s the creation of the Board of Trustees to encourage industry helped the expansion of linen, which became Scotland's most significant industry and of particular significance to Dundee. The bounty on export of coarse linen enabled Dundee to enlarge the market for her industries in her province.[20]

Political developments were not all beneficial. Glasgow had to spend considerably in 1715 in preparing to resist the Jacobite army, and in 1745 avoided looting by the Highland army at the cost of £5,000 sterling. All the same she found resources for new enterprises. Her illegal tobacco enterprise meant that her firms were as well capitalised as those of England when the trade was officially opened. To sustain the innovative store system in the Chesapeake she had to enlarge her overland trade as well as her industrial production. Eventually her own new industries, particularly linen and cotton, became of great significance. In the eighteenth century she became an exceptionally busy city, with a small and not very rich middle class. There were not many professional men; it was the business world that dominated. The readiness of Glaswegians to start up new industries led to expansion beyond the system of guilds. She was marked for the many societies geared to benevolence, and also to social life. It was in the universities of Glasgow and Aberdeen that the Scottish Enlightenment first came to life. In 1783 another sign of enterprise was the creation of the first British Chamber of Commerce.[21]

The general expansion of the large towns is marked by their population increase. Webster's census of 1755 gives Edinburgh and her satellites 57,195 inhabitants, Glasgow 23,546, the two Aberdeens together 15,436, and Dundee 12,477.[22] These figures should be regarded merely as approximations. They indicate increases respectively on the 1690s of 110 per cent, 65 per cent, 62 per cent and 35 per cent. Edinburgh's expansion is partly a sign of increased government, but it also reflects the rapid growth of South Leith in the 1740s and 50s resulting from expansion of trade with Europe and England.[23] Glasgow's vigorous growth reflects the rising importance of transatlantic trade.

These towns had had to create extra parishes: the Gorbals was split off from Govan into a separate parish, in Edinburgh Greyfriars was divided between 'Old' and 'New', and by the 1780s Dundee possessed five parishes. New streets were added and new trades and products appeared. Even old products changed. Scottish brewers learnt better formulae and Scottish weavers mastered the art of making softer blankets. In the 1740s all Scottish figures for production or export show a sudden upward movement. Transport had been improving since Union. The post, newspapers and banks were all helpful to enterprise. The birth of what has come to be called consumerism is shown in the commodities that can be found in the inventories of household possessions – better furniture, pictures, implements for eating and drinking, mirrors, clocks and luxury fabrics. Some of these objects were imported, but rapidly the towns learnt to manufacture them themselves.[24]

The big towns followed the European movement for the provision of recreation. The Directory of Edinburgh for 1752 shows new features which manifest this.[25] There were six coffee houses, many more goldsmiths, apothecaries, milliners and mantua makers than in the past, and 56 households engaged in some part of book production. The city council had been investing in expanding the university and bringing in new subjects for lecture courses as a means of enticing foreign students, particularly those from England. Gentry families could come from the country and get schooling and tutoring for their children.

The removal of the centre of ambitions of the great lords to London after Union, where jobs and power would be found, had liberated the gentry from oppression, and allowed them freedom of expression. The ability of the Church to repress activities that it did not approve of had drastically weakened. 'Promiscuous dancing' had long been the object of its denunciation, but a small and soberly conducted Assembly Room had opened in Edinburgh in the 1740s and was followed by larger successors. The magistrates successfully prevented a theatre company being set up in the 1720s, but they could not stop visits by companies, and in the 1750s a regular season of plays started up. Music, for those who could pay a high subscription, had been available since the 1720s.[26] Outside recreations used the space of Leith. There was a regular summer week of horse racing on the Links there, interfered with only by the tide, and a golf course. There was even a single bathing machine on the shore.[27]

A recent study of Edinburgh has claimed that social division in location and patterns of recreation became more marked after 1730: the richer part of the city's population separated itself from the rest, geographically as well as in economic function, and it was to this part that the new recreations and cultural activities were restricted. Certainly the building of the new town a generation later led to some social separation, but the new town had its own service areas, occupied by tradesmen. It is also clear that in the world of religion, whether within the established church or in dissent, a considerable amount of power lay with people who were not of the social elite.[28]

The other towns followed the same policy of creating facilities with which to attract the gentry of their regions, though Dundee was relatively backward. Mid-century the town is described not as a 'one horse town' but as a 'one chaise town'. Her rural aspect was shown by the lack of slated roofs and by the habit of the women of keeping shoes for wear only on Sundays.[29] But Dundee, already expanding, grew sharply in the transformation of Scotland in the third quarter of the century. Its population almost doubled between the 1750s and the 1790s; Aberdeen's went up by over half, Edinburgh's by two thirds and Glasgow's multiplied by nearly three. Edinburgh and Glasgow created their 'new towns' in and after the 1770s, tranquil residential suburbs for the better off, to accommodate some of their growth, and this made them very different from the mixed social pattern of earlier times. It is in this third quarter of the century that we can call the large towns cities.[30]

It was a period when Scotland was transformed. Change was particularly marked in the cities. There were four separate and interacting strands in the changes which led to Scotland becoming a modern and urbanised society. First there was her sensational intellectual achievement in the Enlightenment. This movement, not only European in scale but also embracing the Americas, was a new way of looking at the world, in particular bringing argument and criticism to bear on the institutions of religion and society. Its special area of interest was the study of different types of economy and society and the implications of this for types of government, but it also made its mark in philosophy, economics, history, geology and physics. Its relationship to established religion was ambivalent. Almost all of its participants accepted the revelation of religion in Christianity and the expectation of an after life, while refusing to accept the Church's puritanism and distrusting the evangelical revival. Many of the participants in Enlightenment thinking in Scotland were clergy, and this includes most of the university professors who led the way in various fields.[31]

The intellectual movement started in the universities of Aberdeen and Glasgow and spread to Edinburgh. It was sustained by lawyers and by some of the gentry who participated in the clubs and meetings in which the new ideas were expressed, and bought the books that expressed the intellectual conclusions.[32]

Enlightenment thought stopped its criticism short of the basic economy and society which supported its participants. Thinkers took for granted the different ranks of society, the ownership of land and privileges which its members enjoyed, and the limitations on women's legal rights. This conservatism prevented conflict with established opinion. Gentlemen in touch with the new currents of thought could feel pride in their country's position in the intellectual world.

There was a genuine streak of humanitarianism within the movement, and some aspects of this have a close relation to our subject. Criticism of the public rebuking of women for sexual irregularities occurs in the press in the 1750s and can be attributed to Enlightenment thought, as also may be the fact that judges were becoming uneasy over the presumption of murder attached to concealment of any unmarried pregnancy which ended with the death of a baby. But others besides enlightened thinkers shared in the humanitarian movement. Landowners, whatever their religious or intellectual opinions, helped their parishes and shires to make the poor law work in times of food shortages. It became difficult to believe that in as short a time ago as 1696 the Edinburgh ministers had secured execution for blasphemy.[33]

The second important 'modern' feature of late eighteenth-century Scotland was the rise of dissent. The revolution period had produced a significant breach in the idea of a single national Church with the separation off of the episcopalian community. Many of its members were of Jacobite sympathies but those who could accept the coming Hanoverian dynasty were granted toleration for their meeting houses in an Act of 1712. It was to these that English families present in Scotland as part of the assimilation of the government of the country to that of England (for instance, the higher customs officials) would attend. Over time the episcopal church gathered into its membership much of the land-owning class, those who liked orderly services and familiar prayers, and did not relish undergoing two 50-minute sermons in a bare parish church every Sunday.

There was already a core of small scale dissenting groups, a few Quakers in and around Aberdeen, old meeting houses of congregationalists elsewhere. Then in 1733 the Original Secession, a breakaway group of ministers from the established Church who would no longer tolerate the established Church's acceptance of lay patronage in the appointment of ministers, became the first of a series of dissenting presbyterian organisations. It was not a big community; its long term significance was in showing the potential for schism within presbyterianism. Its appeal was austerely to the 'holier than thou' part of the population, and the efforts of such people to achieve a society of saints led to further fragmentation within the organisation.

The Original Secession was followed in 1761 by the Relief Church, also in opposition to lay patronage, but less determined on separation. It was the function of the Relief Church to offer shelter for congregations temporarily at issue with their minister or patron, congregations which might later return to the establishment. Between them these two communions may have housed a noticeable part of the population of the cities. We have no reliable figure, but somewhere between 10 and 25 per cent seems likely by the 1770s, and growing. The extremely cordial relationship of the established Church with its neighbour Relief church was commented on in relation to Dundee in the 1770s, and it is clear from Glasgow kirk session records toward the end of the century that co-operation rather than rivalry characterised the situation there too. However, these developments weakened the hold of the established Church on its own members, who might change their allegiance if disciplined or pressed.[34]

The third strand marking the late eighteenth century was the agrarian transformation of lowland Scotland. Between 1730 and 1760 joint tenancies virtually disappeared from farms in central Scotland, which became separate units, with one tenant. The drastic change after 1760 was the removal of the whole class of cottars from the small holdings that they held on the old farms. Farms were enlarged by this land. Some cottars continued to live on the farm, as labourers, but most moved to nearby villages or made new settlements. Some became surplus labour in their areas and moved to the towns. The biggest layer of the old rural population had been dispersed.[35]

We do not have figures for the number who abandoned the countryside for town life, but given the overwhelming agricultural emphasis of early modern Scotland, it did not need more than a small proportion of the old labour force to shift to the towns to make a vast pool of labour for industry. At last the surplus product of the countryside was large enough to sustain a big industrial sector. The fourth strand was the urban and industrial transformation which used the new labour force.

Scotland's exports increased dramatically after 1750, and there was also a larger market at home.[36] The urban craftsman could now eat with a knife and fork, drink tea from a well made cup and enjoy good quality porter. The luxury purchase of tea became possible even in the countryside. Wages were rising. Towns in general expanded, but the large towns grew phenomenally. In 1755 they had held nearly nine per cent of the country's population; in the 1790s it had become nearly 13 per cent and growing. Scotland was to become one of Europe's most urbanised countries, and it is in the decades after 1750 that it starts the march towards that position.

It is clear from the material that we have gathered that in the 1770s the Church could no longer hope to control the behaviour of the bulk of the people. The evidence from Edinburgh and Aberdeen particularly shows this. Dundee and Glasgow were apparently carrying on the old discipline, but in Dundee there is evidence of cases being missed or evaded. The attitude of much of the more vocal of the public was changing. A stronger individualism prevailed, particularly among men, who were increasingly wishing to decide personal and moral issues on their own. This was not simple anti-clericalism, but more a demand of the right to make one's own decisions within the bounds of the law. The spectrum of dissent offered different types of religious allegiance; the range of careers made for new openings. There seemed less need to conform to established norms.

How could the cities hope to create and maintain a godly community? There was an inevitable tension between the system of social control established after the Reformation (and still working very satisfactorily in rural parishes throughout Scotland) and the rapidly expanding urban areas with their progressive ideas. This clash is the core of our study of 'sin in the city'.

Notes

1 *Register of the Privy Council of Scotland*, Vol. XIII 1622–1627 (Edinburgh, 1895), p. 511.
2 I.D. Whyte, 'Population Mobility in early modern Scotland', in R.A. Houston and I.D. Whyte (eds.), *Scottish Society 1500–1800* (Cambridge, 1989), pp. 1–35.
3 T.M. Devine, 'The merchant class in the larger Scottish towns in the seventeenth and eighteenth centuries', in G. Gordon and B. Dick (eds.), *Scottish Urban History* (Aberdeen, 1983), pp. 92–111.
4 Our information on Aberdeen comes from G.R. DesBrisay, 'Authority and Discipline in Aberdeen, 1700–1750' (University of Aberdeen Ph.D. thesis, 1989).
5 T. Tucker, 'Report on the Settlement of the Revenue of Excise and Customs in Scotland 1656' in Scottish Burgh Record Society, *Miscellany* (Edinburgh, 1881), pp. 1–48.
6 R.E. Tyson, 'The Economy and Social Structure of Old Aberdeen in the Seventeenth Century', in John S. Smith (ed.), *Old Aberdeen: Bishops, Burghers and Buildings* (Aberdeen, 1991), pp. 38–56.
7 *List of pollable persons in the Shire of Aberdeen*, 2 volumes (New Spalding Club, Aberdeen, 1844).
8 Duncan Adamson, *West Lothian Hearth Tax, 1691 with county abstracts for Scotland* (Scottish Record Society, Edinburgh, 1981), p. 96.
9 T.M. Devine and Gordon Jackson (eds.), *Glasgow, vol. 1, beginnings to 1830* (Manchester,

1995), pp. 67–8.
10. James Cleland, *Statistical tables relative to the City of Glasgow* (Glasgow, 1823).
11. Anthony Slaven, *The Development of the West of Scotland 1750–1960* (London, 1975), Chs. 1 and 2; Devine 'The Merchant Class'; T.C. Smout, 'The Glasgow merchant community in the seventeenth century', *Scottish Historical Review* 1968, pp. 53–71; C.O. Oakley, *The Second City* (London and Glasgow, 1945); Devine and Jackson, *Glasgow*, pp. 46, 69–78, 113–14.
12. Helen M. Dingwall, *Late-Seventeenth-Century Edinburgh: a demographic study* (Aldershot, 1994), pp. 21–4; Adamson, *West Lothian Hearth Tax*.
13. Hugh Ouston, 'York in Edinburgh: James VII and the Patronage of learning in Scotland, 1679–88', in J. Dwyer, R.A. Mason and A. Murdoch (eds.), *New Perspectives on the Politics and Culture of Early Modern Scotland* (Edinburgh, 1982), pp. 129–55; T.C. Smout, *Scottish Trade on the Eve of Union* (Edinburgh, 1963), Ch. 11.
14. Dingwall, *Edinburgh*, 27, pp. 289–93, 350.
15. Walter Makey, 'Edinburgh in Mid-Seventeenth Century', in Michael Lynch (ed.), *The Early Modern Town in Scotland* (London, 1987), p. 196.
16. Dingwall, *Edinburgh*, 27, pp. 249–50.
17. Sue Mowat, *The Port of Leith* (Edinburgh, 1994).
18. *List of pollable persons...Aberdeen*, vol. 2, pp. 625–9, 652.
19. Devine, 'The merchant class', 92–111.
20. David Loch, *A Tour through most of the Trading Towns and Villages of Scotland* (Edinburgh, 1778), pp. 26–7.
21. Devine and Jackson, *Glasgow*, pp. 165, 319–42.
22. J.G. Kyd, *Scottish Population Statistics* (Scottish History Society, Edinburgh, 1952).
23. South Leith catechising lists, Scottish Record Office, CH2/716/327.
24. H. Hamilton, *An Economic History of Scotland in the Eighteenth Century* (Oxford, 1963), Chs. 5, 7 and 9, Appendices 3 and 4.
25. J. Gilhooley, *A Directory of Edinburgh in 1752* (Edinburgh, 1988).
26. James H. Jamieson, 'Social Assemblies of the Eighteenth Century', in *The Book of the Old Edinburgh Club*, vol. 19, 1933, pp. 31–96.
27. James Scott Marshall, *Old Leith at Leisure* (Edinburgh, 1976); James Scott Marshall, *The Life and Times of Leith* (Edinburgh, 1986), Ch. 4.
28. R.A. Houston, *Social Change in the Age of Enlightenment – Edinburgh 1660–1760* (Oxford, 1994), pp. 215–27; Richard B. Sher, 'Moderates, Managers and Popular Politics in Mid-Eighteenth-Century Edinburgh: the Drysdale Battle of the 1760s', in Dwyer, Mason and Murdoch (eds.), *New Perspectives*, pp. 179–209.
29. Billy Kay, *The Dundee Book* (Edinburgh, 1990).
30. The figures for the population of the cities in the 1790s are given in the opening pages of the original edition of the *Statistical Account of Scotland*. They are: Edinburgh (with satellites), vol. 6 – 84,886; Glasgow (without Barony), vol. 5 – 61,945; Barony, vol. 12 – 16,451; Govan, vol. 14 – 8,318; Aberdeen (both towns), vol. 19 – 29,493; Dundee, vol. 8 – 21,500.
31. Richard B. Sher, *Church and University in the Scottish Enlightenment* (Edinburgh, 1985).
32. Paul B. Wood, *The Aberdeen Enlightenment* (Aberdeen, 1993).
33. Hugo Arnot, *A Collection and Abridgement of Celebrated Criminal Trials in Scotland* (Edinburgh, 1785), pp. 392–7, The trial of Thomas Aikenhead, 1696.
34. A.L. Drummond and J. Bullogh, *The Scottish Church 1688–1843* (Edinburgh, 1973), Ch. 2; Callum Brown, *A Social History of Religion in Scotland* (Edinburgh, 1987), Ch. 2; Loch, *Tour*.
35. T.M. Devine, *The Transformation of Rural Scotland* (Edinburgh, 1994).
36. T.C. Smout, 'Where had the economy of Scotland got to in the third decade of the eighteenth century', in I. Hont and M. Ignatieff, *Wealth and Virtue* (Cambridge, 1983), pp. 45–72.

2

The Mechanisms of Social Control

In early modern thinking 'sin' and 'crime' were not discrete concepts, the former to come under ecclesiastical jurisdiction and the latter under civil. Parliament passed laws against 'immorality' in the same way as the Church did. After the Reformation the Church demanded that the civil authorities punish fornication, and in December 1564 the Privy Council passed an Act against fornication. A similar Act was passed by Parliament in 1567. Those found guilty faced a fine of forty pounds plus imprisonment for eight days on bread and water and a two-hour public appearance in the mercat place, with higher penalties for repeated offences.[1] The Act remained in force during the centuries that followed but seems to have been enforced only against prostitutes.

In his *History of Church Discipline in Scotland* Ivo Macnaughton Clark argued that 'in many ways the Church's tendency to fall back upon the Civil Magistrates, when her own discipline failed her, undermined what authority she had,'[2] the implication being that at the Reformation some kind of pure ecclesiastical authority existed which was later subverted. However, this is nonsense, for the *First Book of Discipline* incorporated the demand for civil intervention. In a godly society the civil magistrates also had a part to play.

The *First Book of Discipline*, the canon under which the Reformation was established in Scotland, had a heading entitled 'Ecclesiastical Discipline' which concerned the Church's methods of dealing with faults in her members. Such methods were to be preventive in the first instance (public appearances for sins were to be for 'edification'), then remedial and restorative, to win sinners back from error, and finally protective, to guard the 'purity of the Church'. As the original Confession of Faith declared that a godly discipline was one of the signs of a true church, a congregation could not have considered itself part of the true church unless it sustained discipline.[3]

The formal structure for enforcing such discipline was a hierarchy of courts: a kirk session in each parish, a presbytery above it covering a specific region, a synod covering a much larger area (equivalent to a medieval diocese), and finally, at the top, the General Assembly. All ecclesiastical legislation had to be approved by presbyteries before it could be passed by the General Assembly. Between 1660 and 1690 bishops and presbyteries worked together, which made it marginally easier to exert social control over the gentry, as they might be willing to listen to a bishop where they would not listen to a parish minister.[4]

The moderator of a kirk session was the minister; in city parishes with more than one minister the incumbents would take it in turns to officiate. The other session members were known as elders and deacons. According to the *First Book of Discipline* eldership was supposed to be permanent, but in cities we found that elders did not serve for life but had to be re-elected at intervals. Deacons existed in most city parishes as a lower tier. Gordon DesBrisay found that in Aberdeen eighteen elders and eighteen deacons were elected annually. The traditional view of social control in Scottish burghs is that it was carried out by a narrow oligarchy, but DesBrisay emphasised the sheer numbers involved: for 33 of the 44 sessions between 1650 and 1700 he discovered that a total of 1,188 places were filled by 306 men, 62 per cent of whom were merchants and 38 per cent craftsmen. Although a third of deacons went on to become elders, it was clear that 'in essence the two tiers of the church court catered to different sectors of the craft and guild hierarchies.[5] The 'Roll' of the Edinburgh General Kirk Session in the early eighteenth century reveals ex-bailies, advocates, writers to the signet, and gentry amongst the elders, none of which are to be found in the ranks of deacons. The distinction is borne out by the research of R.A. Houston, though he did find some who made the transition from deacon to elder.[6]

In Aberdeen DesBrisay noted that during the episcopal era every session automatically enrolled the seven most senior town council officials – provost, bailies, dean of guild and treasurer – over and above those already elected.[7] Lists of Aberdeen elders in eighteenth century session registers continue to record the presence of provost and bailies. DesBrisay also noted that the Aberdeen eldership was dominated by the same merchants who controlled the town council, and concluded that 'The natural bonds of common interest which already united civic and church leaders were greatly reinforced by the simple expedient of blurring the distinctions between the two groups so as to form what amounted to a single seamless ruling elite.'[8] Meetings of Edinburgh General Session were also attended by the provost and town council. A comparison of elders' names and town council members' names in Dundee in 1755 and 1765 shows that the provost, bailies and magistrates were also elders.[9] However, as will be discussed later, the idea that this automatically meant a 'seamless ruling elite' – or as Stephen Davies put it, that the courts 'shared so many members that they were one body simply "wearing different hats"'[10] – may be something of an oversimplification.

Kirk sessions levied a fine for each offence, though most urban sessions referred this function to the civil authorities. The money would be used to help fund poor relief (for the elderly and disabled) and it is one of the ironies of the system that a more sinful population meant more provision for the needy.

However, the crux of church discipline was not the fine but public appearances to be rebuked before the congregation. For a first fall in fornication the woman and the man had to appear three times, for a 'relapse' six times, for a further fall 26 times. A first offence of adultery would require 26 appearances in sackcloth. For 'antenuptial fornication' – i.e. anticipating the wedding (and having this act betrayed by the early birth of a child) – one appearance usually sufficed. There were, however, local variants on the number of public appearances considered necessary.[11] In 1707, in an attempt to standardise procedures, a new Form of Process was adopted by the Church, and remained nominally in force until 1902.[12] However, as will be seen later, individual kirk sessions were still capable of adopting their own procedures.

Clark comments that the Form of Process was much more legalistic than the First and Second Books of Discipline and the Order of Excommunication of the 1560s. The offender was a 'case' rather than a soul to be won back, if possible, to the fold of Christ.[13] The fundamental difference between the sentences of secular courts and ecclesiastical courts was supposed to be that the former were purely punitive while

2: The Mechanisms of Social Control

the latter were also meant to be redemptive. The extent to which kirk sessions fulfilled this role will be looked at later in the chapter, but for now we turn from the ecclesiastical courts to the secular.

Unlike the Church, which established a unified system after the Reformation, the structure of civil authority evolved piecemeal over centuries. William Mackay Mackenzie commented that 'variety and individuality' were 'the dominant notes of burghal administration.' A committee investigating this in 1793 found only two or three burghs at most carrying out town council elections according to Acts of Parliament. Another report, in 1835, after an Act of Parliament had fruitlessly attempted to lay down precise rulings on local elections, concluded: 'from local influences, which it would be vain to attempt to trace, the constitutions of burghs royal... came to exhibit an endless variety in their details'. After describing the complicated system used to choose Edinburgh town council members, R.A. Houston concluded on the one hand that 'the merchants and their allies could, and did, play fast and loose with the city's constitution for political ends', but on the other, 'it did try to run the city in the interests of the bulk of the established inhabitants.'[14]

All burghs had in common a town council with overall responsibility for the burgh, and from which the civil courts emanated. In Edinburgh, by the late eighteenth century, the town council consisted of 33 men, though it was the 'ordinary' council of 25 men who carried on the day to day business. The council was composed of two bodies of men, merchants and tradesmen; they were elected, in part, by members of the fourteen incorporations, and partly they chose their own successors.[15] In Aberdeen the council consisted of 17 merchant burgesses and two craft deacons, all elected at Michaelmas for one-year terms of office. As with kirk sessions, DesBrisay commented on the sheer number of men who governed Aberdeen in the late seventeenth century: [the] town council was reconstituted 51 times between Michaelmas 1649 and Michaelmas 1699, each time with a somewhat different cast of characters.[16]

The most important members of any town council were the magistrates and bailies. Hugo Arnot commented in the late eighteenth century: 'The magistrates of Edinburgh are vested with ample powers, and an extensive jurisdiction; a jurisdiction which they formerly exercised in a latitude not to be paralleled but in a despotic monarchy; a latitude which has never been circumscribed by positive law, but alone by the imperceptible operation of the prevailing principles of liberty.'[17]

In Edinburgh burgh courts, the largest number of cases were petty thefts, followed by prostitution (frequently combined, as in 'common whore and thief'). It was not only women who were taken up on 'morality' charges. For example, in May 1687 Thomas Anderson, indweller in Edinburgh, 'who hes bein within the tolbooth of this burgh for the space of ffyve months or thereby for haunting with debaucht company such as vagabonds and Idle persones who walked on the street under Cloud of night... obleidged himselfe never to be sein in any such company hereafter under the penalty of being scourged throw the toun and banished the same.'[18]

Edinburgh also had a Justice of the Peace Court. JPs were a comparatively recent innovation, dating back only to 1609, though revived by Cromwell in 1655, and they never had the full range of powers of their longer established English equivalents. In the late eighteenth century Arnot commented that while subsequent acts extended their range of activities, these powers were 'not so well understood, nor so accurately defined in Scotland, as in England.'[19] But Houston feels that the JP court 'performed an important integrative function in the Edinburgh area and helped undermine certain lesser jurisdictions.' The minute books bear out his contention that it handled 'a range of cases, some of which had been appropriate to baronial courts.'[20]

The usual sentence for miscreants was to be whipped through the town and then banished. The tolbooth was used mainly for short-term imprisonment, but Edinburgh's 'correction house' was utilised as a long-stay prison. An extreme case was that of Helen Mackenzie, 'ane Common Whore', who had been imprisoned in the tolbooth for five months before appearing before the burgh court in September 1693, after 'haveing often tymes petitioned the Baillies and Kirk session to sett her at Libertie by reasone of her stearving conditione'. The Bailies liberated her on condition that she never be seen in the city again, otherwise 'she shall be brunt on the Cheek & Scourged thorrow the toun Doucked in the north loch and sent to the Correction house to remayn for ever.' How many such sentences were inflicted cannot be known, as the surviving records, the 'enactment books' deal with those who avoided them by promising to leave the burgh.

As mentioned in the previous chapter, Canongate, now a part of Edinburgh, was until 1856 a separate burgh of regality, although the superiority was held by Edinburgh.[21] The Canongate 'Black Books' are similar to those of the Edinburgh burgh court, with thieves and whores predominating. Women who 'can give no Account of themselves or their way of living' were promptly banished. Canongate did not have recourse to the Edinburgh correction house, but it had its own prison and otherwise the punishments inflicted were the same.[22]

Another separate barony (now part of Edinburgh) was Portsburgh, a burgh of barony which lay immediately south of the 'ports' (gates) of the city, and which overlapped much of St Cuthbert's (West Kirk) parish. The magistrates of Edinburgh had the right to choose the bailies and other officers.[23] In December 1704 St Cuthbert's kirk session, 'considering the great loss they sustain through the want of a prison', recommend that the moderator and the Baron of Portsburgh 'speak to the Lord Provost of Edinburgh in order to gett one built'. Reference is made in later Portsburgh baron court records to imprisonment, so presumably the session was successful. Portsburgh had recourse to the Edinburgh correction house. The majority of cases were once again petty theft. A number of individuals bound themselves to keep the peace, and keepers of 'bad' houses also came before the court.[24] Leith was also a burgh of barony for which Edinburgh as superior had the right to choose bailies and other officers and make regulations. Whores do not appear in Leith court records, which is puzzling as South Leith kirk session registers (January, May and July 1661, December 1666, September 1667) mention whore houses.[25]

As noted in the last chapter, the other towns in Scotland had much smaller populations.[26] However, the ability of burghs to establish their own individual systems is vividly illustrated by Aberdeen. When Cromwell revived the idea of Justice of the Peace courts in 1655 Aberdeen seized on this to create a secular equivalent to the kirk session, the justice court. There was also a burgh court, which heard a wide variety of cases, but morality cases were shared between kirk session and justice court.[27] Thus an individual delated to the session for fornication, antenuptial fornication, or adultery would also have to appear before the justice court, and vice versa (the initial delation might be to either court). The justice court fined the offenders – or inflicted corporal punishment on the few who were unable to pay – while the session ordered them to make their public appearances before the

2: The Mechanisms of Social Control

congregation. DesBrisay thought that 'the reason why Aberdeen, seemingly alone among Scottish burghs, found it necessary to maintain two separate judicatories for the same offenders for the same offences stemmed from a local insistence upon the strict separation of secular and ecclesiastical discipline.'[28]

Having looked at the secular side of the picture, we turn back to kirk session records to observe the interaction with civil authorities. In January 1661 there was a spate of referrals to magistrates by Canongate kirk session. On the 8th of the month the elders and deacons were 'desired to search their respective quarters, for scandalous persones and give their names to the magistrats that they may be removed from the parish.' A week later two women, one of whom had been in the correction house, were referred to the magistrates, as was a man 'for resetting [receiving] of papists', and two additional women 'for their scolding and abuseing one another'. A fortnight later 'Alexr Mcbaith workman confessing his sin of drunkenness and cursing he is referd to the magistrats for his punishment', while William Bruce was 'delaited for receiving infamous persones' and when he confessed that one Barbara Strachan 'haunts sometymes his house for drink' he was referred to the magistrates.

This level of interaction between a session and the civil authorities was unusual outside Aberdeen and did not long persist in the Canongate. More typically there was a specific reason for a referral. For example, in January 1663 Walter Hay compeared before Edinburgh St Cuthbert's session '& confessed he wryt ane false testimoniall at the desyr of Bessie Riddoch'. He 'was referred to the civill magistrat being more criminal than ecclesiastick'. A woman suspected of infanticide would normally be referred.[29]

If a session did not believe a woman's accusation of the man who fathered her child they might utilise the civil authorities. In South Leith in March 1661 Isobell Gibb named an Englishman unknown in the parish and was 'referred to the civil magistrats to verifie her bairns father.' In Canongate, April 1663, Christian Kaiplie named a member of the gentry, James Lumsden of Balquhanie, and was 'referd to the magistrats till she verifie her childs father'. (In September he confessed that he was indeed the father.)

Partly the fear was that if there was no man taking on some of the financial responsibility, a session might have to draw on the poors' funds to help the mother. In South Leith, in May 1706, the session learned that Lambart Johnson, named by Janet Ballantine as father of her child, was 'to goe away with the fleet and denys to mantain the Child'. The session applied to the Edinburgh magistrates to bring him under caution 'to free this place of the Burden of the child.' In Canongate a young woman who had borne twins to David Smith, officer of excise, was destitute in April 1748, as 'the said Smith would contribute Nothing to the Relief and Maintenance of the said Children, so that they would become a Burden to the parish.' The session applied 'to a justice of the Peace for a Warrant to bring the said Smith before him and oblige him to find Security to the Care of the said Children and that they should not become a Burden on the Session.' As late as January 1799 in Dundee, Margaret Stewart said that the father of her child was at present in London, 'but refused to tell his Name or expose him... The Moderator and B[aillie] Smith were appointed as a Committee to prosecute her before the Magistrates in order to oblige her to find a security for the Maintenance of her Child.'

Clearly the civil powers were being used to put pressure on individuals. This is made explicit in some instances. In Edinburgh Trinity College (August 1665) Grisell

Maxwell named one Thomas Scot as father. The session did not believe her story and referred her to the magistrates 'to the end they might see what some little times imprisonment might produce'. (A week later she named another man, a member of the gentry, who subsequently confessed guilt.) When Helen Reid appeared before Dundee session in December 1771 she 'refused to tell who the Father thereof was unless the session would inform her whom it was that had raised a bad report upon her since she came to this place – But upon hearing that she was to be put in prison declared that James Dickson an unmarried man belonging to the Excise was the father thereof.' (As she had been pregnant when she arrived in the parish the session thought she should be removed and applied to the provost 'to have her put out of Town with all convenient speed'.) Also in Dundee, in August 1775, when Anne Wilson was delated as being with child, 'being sent for refused to come – The Session having complained to a civil Magistrate she was brought before the session by a Town Officer... Being then asked who was the Father of it answered that it was time enough to know that & for some time after refused to give any other answer till she understood that she was to be sent to Prison'. She then told the session that it was William Macnab, a soldier who had left the parish. (But this was a lie: a year and a half later, when the true father of her child was to marry another woman, she revealed his name.)

One of the two main reasons that sessions made use of civil authorities was because individuals were recalcitrant (the other reason was because they were considered 'not a fit object of church discipline'). Many examples could be given. Indeed, in March 1681 Edinburgh St Cuthbert's sessions 'takeing to their serious consideration the great contempt of the discipline of the Church by the delinquents refusing to compeir upon the ordinar citations till they be compelled by the Civill Magistrat Have therefore with ane consent inacted That what ever delinquents shall conteme the three ordinarie citations shall be fyned in double of the ordinarie penaltie.' In Glasgow Barony in January 1730, the session asked the presbytery's advice on how to compel confessed fornicators to make their public appearances and were told they 'should crave the assistance of the Civil Magistrate in order to cause them give Satisfaction to the Church'.

Sessions also utilised the services of the civil authorities in relation to irregular marriages. In Edinburgh Old Kirk, February 1707, Thomas Wait, jeweller, admitted he was irregularly married to Margaret Wright, but refused 'to make knowen who maried him, where they were maried, when or who wer witnesses thereto And caried very unbeseeminglie and haughtilie before the Session.' He was judged contumacious and referred to the civil magistrate, 'And he being present took him into Custodie'. (Wait produced the marriage certificate and witnesses a month later.) In Edinburgh New Kirk, December 1717, Mary Drysdale and James Caskie 'obstinately refused to compear befor the Session for owning and instructing their Marriage', so they were referred to the magistrates. (Caskie appeared before the session in April, Drysdale in September.)

As mentioned earlier, in Aberdeen the justice court duplicated the kirk session's functions. Gordon DesBrisay found that in the period he looked at – 1650 to 1700 – some 80 per cent of cases appeared before both courts.[30] Looking at fornication cases in the period immediately after his, 1701–5, we found that 84 per cent appeared before both courts. Spot checks showed that in 1720 ten cases appeared before both, six before the justice court only and none solely before the kirk session; in 1730 nine appeared before both courts, seven before the justice court only and three before the session only; in 1740 eight appeared before both, one each before the justices and session; in 1750 eight before both, five before justices only, and two before session only. What is surprising is not the high number appearing in both, since the avowed intent of the justice court was to be responsible for the civil punishment of morality cases, but the cases which appeared in only one of the courts. Couples appearing before the justice court had to produce cautioners that they would satisfy church discipline, so why did some of the names never appear in the kirk session register? Some may have been banished as undesirables, but surely not all. And how did some couples who confessed guilt before the kirk session manage to avoid ever appearing before the justice court? We do not have an explanation to offer.

The justice court took on some of the functions of magistrates in other cities. In November 1740 Alexander Reid confessed fornication and 'band & Enacted himself That in case the said Isobel Man shall bring furth a living Child Then & in that case the Town and freedom of Aberdeen shall be Indemnified and keeped free of the Maintenance & aliment of any such Child under the penalty of ten pounds sterling'. In November 1750 Daniel Mowat similarly enacted himself for the maintenance of Margaret Brechin's child.

However, Aberdeen kirk session also utilised magistrates at times. In June 1736, when the justice court was still going strong, Daniel Campbell, named by Helen Allan as father of her child, denied guilt. She produced witnesses to his admitting paternity, but Campbell refused to compear again. The session therefore appointed 'an Extract hereof to be laid before the Magistrates to whom they refer both Parties & the Witnesses.' In October 1755 Margaret Anderson named Mr George Alexander as father of her child. He denied the charge. She subsequently 'produced an Extract from the Baillie Court' stating that she had named George Chisholm as father before that court in August.[31] The mid-1750s saw the breakdown of the justice court, and it appears that the bailie court was to some extent taking over its role in morality cases.

Aberdeen may have had a unique system, but Edinburgh had semi-autonomous individuals, the kirk treasurers, who were apparently appointed by the town council. In July 1693 Edinburgh general session considered a recommendation by the presbytery, 'bearing that great prejudice hes arisen to the church and particular reflections thereupon By reason that the several kirk Thesrs of this cities doe exact the civill penaltie from scandalous persons without delating them to the several sessions'. In March 1695 the committee appointed for this purpose recommended:

> That when a secret sin comes to the knowledge of the kirk Thesaurer or any one Elder where testimony cannot be brought to prove it That in that caice they are not obliged to make a delation thereof But where a scandall comes to their knowledge that is not secret but may be proven Especiallie when a woman unmaried is with child or hath born a child in such caices it is hereby ordered that they do declare the same to the kirk session to which it belongs or they would be guiltie of concealing open wickedness and scandals.

However, in February 1701, amongst the 'overtures' to be presented to the magistrates was the following: 'That the Kirk Thesr may be discharged from making privat composition for the fynes for publick scandals, and vices, which come Judiciallie Before the Magistrat, or Session, particularlie, That when any Woman Being with chyld, confesseth to him, And delateth the person to whome it is,

Sin in the City

he doe not privatlie Transact, But bring the Woman under caution or secure her till she be Brought Before the Session or Magistrat'.

Yet kirk treasurers continued such practices. In February 1724 the session of St Cuthbert's, which was not an inner city parish, was particularly angry because the kirk treasurer exacted fines 'from persons not guilty in the city, but in this parish'. In Canongate, in May 1729, the session had heard that Mary Seton 'was about to be carried off from this place', so they directed the kirk treasurer 'to use all proper means for preventing the said Mary Setons being carried off and obligeing her to compear before this Session to make her judicial Confession of the Scandal she is charged with, and of the party guilty with her that the same may be purged according to the Rule of this Church.' Mary was imprisoned but later freed by one of the bailies, on the basis of a declaration by the kirk treasurer that she had paid her fine to him. The session was furious, for 'the further Exercise of Church Discipline in this Case is at present stopped, and effectually interrupted And also the interest of the poor of this parish exceeding much injured And all this by the order and Management of the above Baillie & Kirk Thesr of Edinburgh.'

As late as 1738 Christian Spence appeared before St Cuthbert's session and declared 'That she has brought furth in uncleanness three children, one of Sir Alexr Murray of Melgum, the second & third now in her arms are to Mr Edmiston, Skipper in Leith, that they were all three brought furth in Edinr – That she was never call'd before any Church Court, or has made any satisfaction for these repeated uncleannesses, but that the kirk Thesr was satisfy'd'.

Co-operation between ecclesiastical and civil authorities has been a keynote of the chapter, but magistrates did not always accede to session's demands. In 1719 when some individuals who were irregularly married refused to compear before Edinburgh Trinity College session they were referred to the magistrates as contumacious. But on 28 January 1720 the bailie advised the session that 'he could not by Law Oblige them to compear'.

Stephen Davies ascribes the breakdown in the close relationship between local courts to the abolition of heritable jurisdictions (the system under which local landowners inherited the offices of sheriff etc.):

> 1747 was certainly an important watershed. Under the old system, particularly before 1707, a network of interrelated courts existed, each performing a well defined role and supporting the others... This system had slowly become moribund... When the heritable jurisdictions were abolished, the old, localized system was finally destroyed: the local courts disappeared and the church courts were cut off from their most enthusiastic secular supporters and left to 'wither on the vine'.[32]

This analysis seems far less relevant to cities, but it was well after that supposed watershed date that a major row broke out in Dundee. In November 1759 the provost, George Yeaman, demanded that the session's registers of baptisms and marriages be turned over to him. The moderator, Mr Carmichael, refused to do so and was fined ten pounds 'for contumacy'. The session approved the moderator's actions, for the registers were 'in every Respect the property of the session, bought at first with their money, wrote by their servant, according to their orders & directions, the proper Records of their Court'. A committee was appointed 'to draw up a full Memorial of this Matter, & without Delay to transmit the same to an able Lawyer at

Edinburgh, that they may have his advice & counsel upon the whole.'

On the 21st the session learned that 'the Town Council had elected Mr James Greig to be precentor and Keeper of the Registers of Baptisms & Marriages, and ordered him to officiate and uplift the ordinary Dues, contrary to the Sessions Right, and all precedents in this place.' On 13 February (1760) the committee reported that 'they had obtained a Suspension against the Magistrates & Council, respecting the Keeping of the Registers of Baptisms & Marriages'. In September of that year provost Yeaman intervened in the matter of an irregular marriage, telling the couple there was no need for them to appear before the session.

But in November the town council made overtures of peace. The session replied that they were 'far from taking Pleasure in contending with the Magistrates & Council, nay it would give them the highest pleasure, to see all differences done away, in the most speedy and amicable manner.' However, the session was certainly not willing to 'yield up the Rights and privileges, which belong to them as a Society, nor allow these to be taken from them without proper Remonstrance.' If the magistrates and town council would 'leave the Kirk session in the quiet and peaceable Possession of the Rights contended for, and which by Law & Custom, belong to the Session', grant reparation for the injuries sustained by the session and Mr Carmichael, and refund to the session the expenses incurred,

> the Session will rejoice in so happy an End of this Contention, and on their part all former ground of Complaint shall be forgotten. But if the Magistrates and Town Council are not so disposed, the session are sorry to say it... that there will be a Necessity for their going on, without delay, to seek Redress in the way they have begun.

The Council were 'not sensible of their having taken from the Kirk session any of the Rights to which they are by Law entitled'. So the case went on to the Court of Session.

In November 1761 that Court found that 'the Magistrates & Town Council of Dundee have the sole Right of Electing the precentor of the East Church of Dundee But find that the Kirk session have the sole Right of electing the Session Clerk, & that he is entitled to the keeping of the Records of the Baptisms and Marriages and to give Extracts therefrom, and to the Dues of such Extracts, but find that the Fees in use to be given when application is made for proclamation of Banns, belong equally to the precentor and Session Clerk of the East Church of Dundee'. The session appealed against the last part of that decision, and on 24 February 1762 the Court found that 'the Precentor has no Title to any Share of the legal Dues accustomed to be paid to the Session Clerk for proclamation of Banns But that the same belong to the Session Clerk.' Furthermore, in November, the Lords Ordinary found it proved that the actions of the magistrates of Dundee, and particularly of the provost, George Yeaman, against the deceased Mr Carmichael and the kirk session of Dundee had been arbitrary and oppressive. The defenders were found liable for damages and expenses which were 'not to be paid out of, or made a Burden on the Funds belonging to the Town of Dundee, but to be paid by the Defenders themselves personally; and in respect that the Illegal Acts above mentioned have been mostly committed by the Defender provost George Yeaman, finds that he must relieve the other Defenders of the Damages and Expenses awarded to the pursuers by this Interlocutor.'[33]

Sin in the City

Clearly in this instance it was one person who initiated hostilities, but it demonstrates that by this date at least, the fact that town council members were also elders was no guarantee of harmony.

In South Leith in August 1754 the session was trying to locate Helen Wilson, who was said to be with child, and cited a woman who apparently knew where she was. The latter 'absolutely refused to compear, or give any satisfaction in the matter of Helen Wilson', so she was referred to the magistrates 'for securing her Compearance'. On 22 August it was 'Reported from the Magistrates, That having advised with their Assessor they found it incompetent for them to interpose their Authority for compelling Magnus Bayne's Wife, or any other Person, to compear before the Session to give Evidence in Matters of Scandal.' Even in Aberdeen, where, as has been seen, the relationship between the two authorities was particularly close, something similar occurred. William Cruickshank had been seen in the act of fornication with Agnes Ritchie and was cited in May 1750. He ignored citations, and in June the session applied to magistrates to oblige him to attend the session: 'their Answer was, that they would not meddle in the Affair, but that the session might proceed against him according to the Rules of the Church'.

However, there was one thing that ecclesiastical and civil authorities were as united on at the end of the eighteenth century as they were in the middle of the seventeenth, and that was their detestation of whores and brothels. Edinburgh town council passed a law against brothel keepers, pimps and harlots in 1560, and the Privy Council passed a similar act in 1564; the only difference was that Edinburgh ordained that the third fault should be punished by death (though it seems extremely unlikely that this was ever carried out).[34] William Creech's virtuous picture of an Edinburgh containing only five or six brothels in the 1760s, which he sent to the Statistical Account, will not stand up to investigation.[35]

Edinburgh burgh court act books ('Black Books') are full of cases like the following of 2 February 1687:

> The said day... Compeared Anna Drummond & Marion Arthur who hes bein Imprisoned thir severall dayes bygones as common whores and hes bein severall tymes enacted in the black book formerly as notorious whores Theirfore the magistrats ordaines the saids whores to be caryed doun to the correction house and there remaine for the space of seven years.

Or this one of December 1740:

> Isabell Philp a common whore who has been in the Correction house for her bad practises and under sentence of banishment and Margaret Hamilton... who has been formerly in the guard for bad practices Judicially enact themselves furthwith to depart this City and priviledges never hereafter to be seen therein under the pain of being apprehended & committed to the house of Correction & Whipt through this City once every quarter for Seven Years and dureing that time fed upon the expence of their own labour.

It is not only women who appeared in this context. In December 1762 William Knight admitted that he 'has kept a disorderly house in this City for some time past, on which account he was banished some years ago and went to the Canongate, from whence he was also banished on the same account'. He undertook to depart on 'pain of being confined to the house of Correction for twelve months whipt once every three months & again banished.'[36]

Whores and bawdy house keepers also appeared before the Edinburgh JP court. In July 1730 it was reported that Margaret Wright alias Mrs Kirkwood, who had previously been publicly whipped through the city and banished 'for sundry vile and abominable practices... had of late returned to this place and taken up her residence, and assumed a false name, and according to her former practice keeped a baudy house'. (She was again banished under pain of being publicly whipped once a month.) A number of individuals were banished by this court for 'keeping bad houses in this town and entertaining of whores and mixt Companys of men & women & disorderly persons therein to the disturbance of the neighbourhood'. The disturbance of the neighbourhood was perhaps the reason why these cases came before a court dedicated to keeping the peace rather than before the burgh court. It was this aspect which also featured in most complaints that came before kirk sessions. For example, in January 1725 Margaret Carruthers (Mrs Pagan) and her daughter, Jean Pagan, were both accused before South Leith session of keeping bad houses. A witness declared that:

> frequently he has heard a noise of Company in Mrs Pagans house at very unseasonable hours, And particularly upon the night after the 8th Instant, he was much disturbed & raised out of his Bed by rude company that had been in her house, & were seeking to be in again, & calling for the Baudy house, & for the whore Jean Pagan with the red stripped gown And that he heard her frequently Imprecat Curses upon her Neighbours, And That his Daughter being sick, & lying within hearing of the noise of Rude company Cursing & Swearing in Mrs Pagans house, was oblidged to remove her Bed to another part of the house, to be free of the Noise.

What about the men who frequented such places? In June 1736 a complaint was laid before Edinburgh JP court against Robert Alderslie, 'student of Physick residenter in Edinburgh' that he 'had been in a Constant Course and tract of frequenting and haunting Badhouses in and about the City and Committed the vile and abominable act of uncleanness & fornication with women therein and more particularly that yesternight or this morning he was in the house of Mrs Jamieson a person habit and repute for keeping a bad house and there with a woman therein named Mary McLaren a person reputed a Common whore Did committ the said act of uncleanness'. Alderslie was fined 'one hundred pounds Scots money One half thereof payable to the Kirk Treasurer for the use of the poor and the other half to the Fiscalls of Court'. However, for a man to be fined was a rare occurrence.

In a case before North Leith kirk session in November 1737 William Stirling, John Hume and a third man had been found in an Edinburgh bawdy house on a Sabbath. They had apparently disturbed a gentleman living on the floor above, who had gone for the guard who found the three men 'sitting on one side of the Room and four women on the bed side on the other side with their plaids on the bed'. Stirling told the session that neither he nor Hume 'knew any thing of the House's character till a party of the City guard came, upon whose coming the women ran into the room where the Defendant and his Company were sitting and that there were no women with them before that time.' The session did not need to pursue this unlikely tale any further since it could nail him on Sabbath breach.

Of course, Edinburgh was not unique amongst Scottish cities in offering sexual services. In Aberdeen Andrew Young, stabler, was delated in September 1689 'for keeping of ane bordell house', and in January 1690 Margaret Webster was delated 'for keeping ane most Lewd and infamous house'. For the most part, the session left such cases to the justice court, but in August 1767 'it was represented by some of the Elders that many lewd women walked the streets of this City by night, and that there were Houses of bad fame keept in the place'. In May 1777 it was represented to the session 'that a most infamous practice is beginning to prevail in this City of Impudent Women walking the streets both in the Evening, and sometimes thro' the whole Night and behaving in a very indecent manner, to the great offence of the Inhabitants and strangers'. That this was only beginning to happen in Aberdeen as late as the 1770s is hardly credible, and all the session could think of to do was to consider the matter further and ask the magistrates 'to interpose their authority to curb this abominable practice in the most effectual manner they think proper'.

The terms 'bawdy' and 'bad' house were used interchangeably, but in fact such establishments ran the gamut from brothels on the one hand to houses of assignation on the other. The most conspicuous entrepreneur in these matters appears to have been one Aeneas McCulloch in Trinity College, an example of the initiative credited to Highlanders migrating to the Lowlands and finding useful economic niches in which to make a living. In July 1712 his house was named as the place where an unmarried pregnant woman lived, and in September of the same year the same location was named for another. The session had ordered an inquiry into the house. But in 1717 in March, and separately in July, the house was again named as the place of conception of illegitimate children. From the way the house was named specifically in all four cases, it was clearly well known. The striking thing is that none of the above women, whose bastards were begotten in a 'bad' house, were called whores or referred to the magistrates.

The absence of effective action over Aeneas McCulloch may be an example of silence in the record when the Church was up against well organised and institutionalised sexual services for the upper class. An unpleasant instance of this occurred in Canongate, April 1743, when a woman presented a complaint that a twelve year old girl, Jean McFarlane, who lodged with her, had been unwillingly procured for sex. The girl 'declared that when she was begging in the Lawn mercat one Marjory Clark came to her, and gave her a half penny, and desired her to go along with her and she would give her an old apron, and so carried her down to Isobell Ivies house in the head of the Canongate, and thereafter gave her some strong ale and caused her to drink it... and thereafter the said Isobell Ivie went out to the mercat and brought in a collop piece of beef and there came in Sir William'. A bowl of wine was brought in and the girl was forced to drink, and she was then raped by Sir William. The session labelled the offence a 'scandalous and heinous Iniquity', and ordered the prosecution of Isobell Ivie before the civil magistrate for expulsion from the town, but made no move against Sir William, whose name was never recorded in full.

Sir William was beyond the scope of discipline because of status and wealth. At the other end of the scale, prostitutes were left alone by the ecclesiastical authorities as beyond redemption. For example, in January 1738 South Leith session was informed that Mary Couts was 'no proper object of Church Discipline, being an Infamous Scandalous person, who hath brought forth several children, & given no account of their Fathers'. She was referred to the magistrates 'That they may Execute the Law, & Expell her the place'. But by February 1740 Mary was not only still there, but also 'again with child in Uncleanness'. She was once more referred to the magistrates 'for Execution of the Law against such a prostitute common strumpet'.

The ineffectiveness of banishment is borne out in various kirk session registers. For example, in December 1710 Edinburgh New Kirk session were informed that James Watt and his spouse kept a bad house 'and that they were Expelled both out of the West Kirk parish and the Canongate parish for the same guilt Therefor they are Referred to the Magistrat to Expell them the City.' The unlikelihood of that action succeeding may be inferred from the following plaintive note in Trinity College session register of July 1703: 'It was Represented to the Session That there are many persons in Edr who have been Banished the Town for Theft, Whooredome, Keeping bad houses and other Miscarriages... And yet are Living in the Town for they... flee from one paroch to ane other, And Testimonials not being sought from them, they live as if they had never been Banished.'

Clearly, while kirk sessions used civil magistrates to buttress their own authority and to deal with individuals considered to be beyond redemption, the system could never have held up for so long if they had relied solely on the civil powers to enforce discipline. The Church had other weapons in its armoury.

One practice which seventeenth century kirk sessions employed – in common with civil courts – was the use of 'caution' (pronounced 'caytion') – i.e. bail. When a man or woman confessed to a sin and promised to appear publicly before the congregation, a friend or relative would stand pledge for them. Knowing that they would incur a financial penalty if the miscreant failed to appear, the cautioner would make every effort to see that they did. In a case that came before Edinburgh New Kirk parish in April 1706, Margaret Hog's cautioner was threatened with prison if he did not reveal the name of her child's father; he caved in to this pressure and revealed it. (The practice of using cautioners died out in the eighteenth century.) If a wrongdoer still did not appear before the congregation – or if they did not even answer the session's citations in the first place – they would be referred to the presbytery. In some cases, simply invoking a higher court was enough to cause a recalcitrant individual to appear. If they did not, the next step was to call out their name from every pulpit within the presbytery area; if this did not suffice then they would no longer be considered members of the Church.

A particularly powerful sanction which the Church possessed was the withholding of baptism from a newborn child. Baptism continued to exert a powerful hold over the populace in the reformed church, indeed a wetnurse would refuse to accept a child who had not yet been baptised. This weapon was significantly blunted after 1690, especially in Edinburgh where there were so many dispossessed Episcopal ministers ready and eager to perform baptisms. Nevertheless, after the Forty Five rising, both Old Aberdeen and Dundee sessions forced men who had taken part to acknowledge their sin of 'unnaturall Rebellion' before their children were allowed baptism.[37]

A variety of other ploys were used by sessions. In Aberdeen in February 1680 the master of apprentice mariner Murdo Macleud promised the session 'to cause him to satisfie the church censure befor he give him up his Indentures'. In South Leith in December 1695 Jean Clatchie, delated for fornication, was living in Edinburgh, and the clothes she left behind her were seized by magistrates until she appeared. (In cases of Sabbath breach officers often confiscated the plaids of guilty women until they appeared before the session.) In March 1700 in Edinburgh St Cuthbert's the banns were being called for James Elder's marriage to Janet Cuthbertson when he confessed fornication with Isobel Cousdon. He was told that 'if he would not give Bond to obey Church discipline, they would stop the proclamatione of his matrimonial Banns'. Jean Cleland was a poor widow in Trinity College parish who confessed to fornication in October 1703; to ensure her public appearances the session withheld her weekly poor law pension.

The final sanction was excommunication. This took two forms. The 'lesser excommunication' meant that an individual was cut off from 'church privileges', i.e. baptism, communion, marriage etc. In fact, anyone who did not satisfy a session as to their penitence would be left to 'lie under the scandal', which was effectively the same as lesser excommunication, without the formal procedure. It was easy enough for a man or woman to express penitence and be re-admitted to the congregation.

The greater excommunication was an altogether more serious and drawn out affair, for an individual was being turned into an outcast. In July 1713 South Leith session recorded the decision of Edinburgh presbytery regarding the case of Alexander Piry, 'some time pin maker in Leith now Messenger at Arms in Edinburgh'. He had been processed for two adulteries and then left Scotland for some time. On his return 'he fell into some of these scandals, after he had made profession of repentance, for his horrid and abominable wickedness, and so mocked God and his people, and shewed his hypocrisie and Impenitence'. Four years earlier the process of the greater excommunication had been commenced against him, 'and much pains has been [taken] to bring him to a sense of his sin not only by private conferences, but has been thrice publickly admonished, and thereafter thrice publickly prayed for, and after much patience, advertisement was given from the pulpit' that if he did not repent he would 'be cut off from the society of the faithfull'. He had not done so and was duly sentenced 'to be excommunicate and shutt out from the Communion of the faithfull debarring him from their priviledges, and in the words of the Apostle to Deliver him over to Satan and thereafter the said Minister is to warn the people that they shun all unnecessar Converse with him'. We cannot know how such a sentence affected individuals; the rich and powerful might have been able to shrug their shoulders, but to be an outcast from one's community must have appeared a horrific prospect to most.

The Church certainly did strive hard to win back souls and, as mentioned earlier, it was the stress laid on penitence that marked the fundamental difference between ecclesiastical and civil discipline, even for the same offences. Civil courts might have dealt more leniently with penitent offenders, but they punished those offenders and that was the end of it. Church courts required those who came before them to understand and repent their offence. As Heinz Schilling put it, 'The delinquent was a sinner whose inner attitude towards his offence and his church sentence was essential for the result of the disciplinary procedure by the church; a connection which was outside the secular interests of state courts.'[38] Of course, it is impossible for any court to know the 'inner attitude' of someone standing before them, a fact recognised by sessions, as in the case of Agnas Wallace (April 1712) when it was reported to Govan session that 'she seems externally at least to be very affected wt her forsaid sin'. But at least to seem penitent was vital.

This emphasis is particularly striking in Aberdeen, where punitive action was left entirely to the justice court, while the session concentrated on the spiritual welfare of the wrongdoers who came before them. No one was allowed to make a final appearance and be absolved until they understood the 'principles of religion' and their own sin. In December 1707 Margaret Black was 'enquired at anent severall plain truths in the common questions of the Catechism, but she could return no answer thereto, but discovered a great deal of gross and dreadful ignorance'. The session were advised by the presbytery that they 'should take much pains' to instruct her, 'and if after all due pains, she be found still remaining grossly Ignorant, and no greater signs of repentance found with her, than are at present, then that she should be left under the scandal, and publick Intimation made before the Congregation of the reasons thereof.' In January 1715 the session found Jean Michy 'very defective in knowledge and seems nowayes to be affected with a sense of her sin, notwithstanding all the pains taken with her for bringing her to both, agreed, considering that she is learning to read, the great means of coming by knowledge' to give her more time. In August it was reported that 'She hath made a considerable advance in knowledge, and in learning to read, besides that she seems truly to be weighted with a sense of her sin'.

Although women were more likely to appear 'ignorant', men were not exempt from the session's strictures. In February 1715 Aberdeen session found that Alexander Farquhar, merchant, 'discovers great unsoundness in the faith by his answers he made to some grave but plain questions proposed unto him... Besides that he seems not to be so weighted with a sense of his sin as becomes a person in his circumstances.' The whole procedure of instruction by means of 'conferences' continued through the eighteenth century, and a man or woman would have to be found 'tolerably knowing and penitent' in order to be absolved. As late as July 1783 the session, on hearing James Angus, adulterer, 'catechised in their presence found him so Grossly Ignorant & so little affected with a sense of his heinous Sin that they were unanimously of opinion, that it would answer No Christian Edification to admit him immediately but as they were willing to shew him all tenderness they appoint him to confer with the Ministers.'[39]

While the consistency of Aberdeen's emphasis on knowledge and penitence is striking, the two Glasgow sessions, Govan and Barony, also took this very seriously. While making his public appearance before Govan congregation in April 1714, James Nimmo was 'exhorted to deall wt God for a spirit of repentance, that so he might get an sight of his sin in its vileness, and so he would be made to abhor, and to humble himself in dust and ashes, as also the minister held furth to him how that by his sin he was excluded from heaven unless by repentance'. Barony elders conferred with Margaret Shaw and Hugh Burns on numerous occasions between July and December 1704 in an attempt to bring them to a sense of their sin, but 'they seemed still to be little affected for all the pains that had been taken upon them both by the minister and elders. The Session... finding that they grow not better by delaying them; They thought it fitt to declare this unto them, that while they remained thus stupid, the session could not but look upon them as persons incapable of partaking of church priviledges'. In August 1708 that session had three men and five women before them who had long been dealt with without success, and advised them that they must all appear publicly the following Sabbath, 'And that it shall be declared to them befor the Congregation, that though they had given thus far outward obedience, yet the Session did find no signs of their being so much as moraly serious, and therefore could not but judge them as persons uncapable of Church priviledges.' Again, this concern did not disappear over time, for in December 1754

Marion Taylor, having made one appearance before Govan congregation, was told to 'mourn for this her sin and all other of her sins and to beg that God would enlighten her understanding and bring her to a saving sense of her sin, and she being found ignorant of the saving knowledge of Christ', was ordered to confer with the minister and elders.

The infrequency with which this is mentioned in other city parishes may mean that the punitive side predominated, or it may simply mean that the necessary procedures were taken so for granted as not to need mentioning. When Jean Brown completed her public appearances before South Leith congregation in August 1695, it was reported that 'she appeared to have a sense of sin upon her and to be moraly serious'; presumably no one would have been absolved if they had not demonstrated these qualities. In Edinburgh Trinity College James Sinclair of Lyth, Clerk to the Bill Chamber, did not appear before the session, but in December 1719 elders reported that they had 'frequently dealt with his Conscience in private in order to bring him to a sense of his sin but notwithstanding of all the pains taken on him this way they cannot bring him to such a sense thereof as that they can absolve him from the scandal'. The fact that they felt this way about a professional man and member of the gentry implies that even in Edinburgh no one would have been absolved until they had convinced a session of their true penitence.

The aim of all sessions was, of course, for the ideology to become internalised, not simply imposed from above. There is plenty of evidence that it did become so. In Aberdeen in January 1721 William Young confessed guilt with a woman who had left the parish and could not be located. The session agreed to allow him to begin his public appearances in view of 'the deep humiliation and sore stress of mind he is under'. In Govan, in October 1722, Isobell Watson after her second appearance was near her time of delivery; it was reported that 'she was very Infirm and apprehensive of Death and very Desirous of absolution.' In 1766 Robert Adam, weaver, came to Barony session of his own accord, acknowledging that he had been guilty of perjury before the JP court, 'for which grievous sin he could get no rest in his Mind untill he should unbosom himself to the session And was willing to undergo discipline therefor'.

Clark wrote that it was very rare for offenders voluntarily to appear to confess their sins before a kirk session,[40] but we found that a significant proportion of women, and a smaller one of men, spontaneously confessed their sexual involvement to their session. The note 'compeared of her own accord' is rare in the seventeenth century, except in the register of South Leith, but it is a persistent feature after 1700. It may be that session clerks did not bother to record it in the seventeenth century, but it seems likelier that the need for absolution became more internalised later. In Glasgow Barony these cases made 17 per cent of all female cases in the 1710s, in Edinburgh St Cuthbert's 14 per cent in the 1730s, in Aberdeen 11 per cent in the 1760s; these were the peak figures. Male self-reporting was less frequent but occurred in all our cities. Self confession did not mean that a sinner got off any part of the formal penance, but it may have made it easier to establish the fact of penitence.[41]

If parishioners had, to some extent at least, absorbed and internalised the values and principles of the church, the obvious question is: why did the system break down? With the exception of the suburban West Kirk parish, it did so earlier in Edinburgh than anywhere else in the country. In Canongate the session decided in

2: The Mechanisms of Social Control

June 1758 to turn the stool of repentance into a pew or seats, which tells its own tale.

Kirk sessions tried to keep undesirables out of their parish by demanding a testificate signed by the minister of the parish from which newcomers had arrived; those without such a testimonial would not be allowed to stay. This worked well in most parishes but not in a big city. In October 1707 Elisabeth Allan appeared before Edinburgh Old Kirk session, accused of keeping a bad house. She was asked if she and her husband had testificates from the parishes where they had previously dwelt; 'she answered they have no testificats neither did they ever seek any for she lived all her days in this City, first in this paroch at the head of Comms Closs, and thereafter in the new kirk paroch And then in the Tron Kirk paroch and last in the horss wynd att the Foot of the Cannongat, And from thence came back to this paroch at whitsunday last.' Maintaining control over such a mobile (and constantly growing) population proved an impossible feat for Edinburgh inner city sessions.

In the whole of Scotland, as the eighteenth century progressed, there was a changing ethos, away from rigid Calvinist fundamentalist theology to 'moderacy'.[42] The protests of humanitarian thinkers which can be seen in the *Scots Magazine* for 1757 and 1777 and elsewhere,[43] and their claim – that the threat of the outrage to female modesty involved in public censure was a cause of concealment of pregnancy and child murder – may well have had influence. A legal process, much publicised in the press, produced in 1776 the judicial statement that 'There may be a liberty of the pulpit in the matter of censure necessary to the improvement of the morals of the congregation, But... clergymen have no right to expose the character and conduct of a particular person', a judgement which struck at the roots of the practice of godly discipline.[44]

One indicator of change was the willingness of a session to accept money in lieu of appearances before the congregation. Old Aberdeen was the earliest urban parish to do this. The first case was an isolated one in October 1744 when Walter Leith, son to the Laird of Threefield, was allowed to be dismissed with a sessional rebuke after paying three guineas for the poor. Nine years later, in July 1753, John Middleton, merchant, 'declared that he was willing to give two guineas to the Poor providing the session would dispense with his publick appearances. The session considering that his publick appearances would not tend much to Edification unanimously agreed to dispense therewith.' In May 1761 Joseph Simpson asked to be dismissed with a sessional rebuke, saying 'he would pay something considerable for the behoof of the poor besides the ordinary penalty.' As 'the scandal had made very little noise in this parish', the session unanimously agreed.

The first time Aberdeen St Nicholas session had this offer made to them – in December 1758 – they took a vote on whether the man should be rebuked publickly or sessionally, 'and Votes marked it carried by a majority for a sessional rebuke.' In July 1765 the session still felt it had to justify allowing Alexander Grant to get away with this; because he was 'a mere Boy' the session agreed to take his two guineas and dispense with his public appearances. When Robert Grieve, candlemaker, proposed, in September 1769, 'to give some money, for the Benefit of the Poor, in proportient his Circumstances, and begged that the session would accept of what he could afford, and dismiss him from Discipline with a sessional rebuke; The Session named Two Guineas as the lowest they would take from him'. By December 1774 the practice had become so common that the price had dropped considerably; at that time the session standardised it at half a guinea.

Sin in the City

It would not be fair to call Aberdeen session mercenary for accepting money in lieu of appearances, since that money did not line anyone's pockets; it was used for the poor. But the basic principle – that church discipline was primarily redemptive rather than punitive – was hopelessly undermined. In December 1775, with the agreement of the magistrates, Aberdeen session drew up a completely new plan of discipline. A church treasurer was to be chosen by the session and approved by the magistrates. He was to have full authority to prosecute (in the session's name) all delinquents 'before the proper Judges, in order to recover from such persons the fines imposed by Acts of parliament and destined for pious uses'. He could accept payment in lieu of appearances and did not need to divulge names. An example of a case that came before the session after that date was Margaret Lawson. In May 1775 the officer reported 'that he had cited her pro 2do that she seemed to make light of the summonds'. In July the treasurer reported that she 'and her party [not named] had given him the satisfaction required, and the process against her is dropt'.

Not all urban parishes went down this road. In Dundee in September 1776 James Watt, periwig maker, 'craved that the Session would be pleased to dispence with his public appearances & rebuke him in private'. The session 'were of Opinion that they could not grant the Request the like having never been granted to any other in this place before.' In Dundee and Glasgow effective church discipline continued to be exerted long after the end of our period.

The fundamental change at this time – a product partly of the new ethos, but also of the growth of dissenting sects offering disaffected members of the established church other congregations to join – was voluntarism. Previously it was believed that every member of the congregation had to be redeemed, not so much for the sake of the individual as for the purity of the congregation. Now the premise was that an unredeemed individual was not a member of the congregation; if that individual wanted to rejoin the communion of the faithful it was up to him or her to apply to satisfy discipline. Margaret Dryborough was asked by North Leith session in November 1768 'if she was willing to make her appearance before the Congregation for her said sin, answered she was, when she should be called upon'. John Hay, appearing before the same session in January 1770, acknowledged himself the father of Grizel Mitchel's child, '& engaged before the session, to maintain and support it. Being asked if he was willing to make public satisfaction for his sin; answered he was not, upon which the Moderator... intimated to him that without his making a public acknowledgment he could not be admitted to partake of church priviledges'. Even in Dundee, public appearances had to be sued for and were not allowed unless the individuals were considered worthy. That session regularly suspended men and women from church privileges; most craved to be re-admitted, but only those whose conduct was considered satisfactory were allowed to do so.

There is irony in the fact that the cities where discipline continued to be powerfully exerted were Dundee and Glasgow, the towns where dissent had the greatest hold. Those who remained within the established church no longer did so because they had no choice but were there because they believed in its tenets; the church's hold over them was therefore stronger than ever. And dissenting congregations offered no refuge from church discipline, as in many cases they were even stricter than the established church. However, the monolithic church structure, which had been able to operate so effectively in tandem with the civil authorities for so much of our period, no longer existed at the end of it.

2: The Mechanisms of Social Control

Notes

Edinburgh, Canongate and Leith kirk session registers are in the Scottish Record Office; the only exception is Edinburgh New Kirk which for the year 1706 is in Edinburgh University Library and for several other years in Edinburgh City Archive. Aberdeen St Nicholas registers are in Aberdeen City Archive; Old Machar registers are in the parish church, with access via Aberdeen University – microfilms of both sessions' records are in the Scottish Record Office. Glasgow Barony and Govan session registers are in Glasgow City Archive, and have not been microfilmed. Dundee registers are in Dundee City Archive, with microfilms in Edinburgh. We have not given references for each citation but always state the month and year, making it possible for anyone to find a particular case.

1. J.R. Hardy, 'The Attitudes of Church and State in Scotland to Sex and Marriage, 1500–1707' (unpublished M.Phil. thesis, University of Edinburgh, 1978), p. 433.
2. Ivo McNaughton Clark, *A History of Church Discipline in Scotland* (Aberdeen, 1929), p. 175.
3. Ibid., p. 26, Rosalind Mitchison and Leah Leneman, *Girls in Trouble: Sexuality and Social Control in Rural Scotland 1660–1780* (Edinburgh, 1998), Ch. 1, in which we spelled out in much more detail the rationale behind church discipline.
4. In *Girls in Trouble* we discussed each of these courts in much greater depth.
5. Gordon Russell DesBrisay, 'Authority and Discipline in Aberdeen 1650–1700' (unpublished Ph.D. thesis, St Andrews University, 1989), p. 310.
6. Each Edinburgh parish had its own session, but there was an additional tier, the General Session, which comprised representatives from all the inner city sessions and passed local statutes. Edinburgh General Session material is in the Scottish Record Office (SRO) CH2/131/2; R.A. Houston, *Social Change in the Age of Enlightenment – Edinburgh 1660–1760* (Oxford, 1994), pp. 200–203.
7. DesBrisay, 'Authority and Discipline', p. 309.
8. Ibid., p. 311.
9. Town Council minutes are in Dundee City Archive.
10. Stephen J. Davies, 'The Courts and the Scottish Legal System 1600–1747: The Case of Stirlingshire', in V.C. Gatrell, Bruce Lenman and Geoffrey Parker, *Crime and the Law* (London, 1980), p. 140.
11. For example, we found that in Trinity College parish in the 1660s unmarried couples who declared that fornication had been committed under promise of marriage had to make just one public appearance, which was not the case in other parishes, since couples did sometimes change their minds after promising. Conversely, in March 1703 Dundee session, 'taking into their serious consideration the abounding sin of antenuptial fornication' ordained that couples guilty of this would have to be rebuked three Sabbaths, 'as fornicators are'.
12. Clark, *A History of Church Discipline*, pp. 142, 148.
13. Ibid., p. 147.
14. William Mackay Mackenzie, *The Scottish Burghs* (Edinburgh and London, 1949), pp. 130–1; Houston, *Social Change in the Age of Enlightenment,* pp. 344–6.
15. Hugo Arnot, *The History of Edinburgh from the Earliest Accounts to the Year 1780* (Edinburgh, 1816), pp. 391–2. Arnot noted: 'Their powers, indeed, and their numbers, have frequently varied; but they now appear to be established beyond the possibility of being altered, but by an act of the legislature.' He went on the describe the extraordinarily convoluted process of electing the town council.
16. DesBrisay, 'Authority and Discipline', pp. 229, 259.
17. Arnot, *History of Edinburgh,* p. 382.
18. Edinburgh Burgh Court Act Books ('Black Books') are in Edinburgh City Archive.
19. Arnot, *History of Edinburgh,* p. 382.

Sin in the City

20 Houston, *Social Change in the Age of Enlightenment*, p. 121. Edinburgh JP Minute Books are in the SRO: JP35/4/2 and 3.
21 Mackenzie, *The Scottish Burghs*, p. 84.
22 Canongate Black Books of Acts are in Edinburgh City Archive.
23 Mackenzie, *The Scottish Burghs*, pp. 83–4.
24 Potsburgh Baron Court Books of Acts are in Edinburgh City Archive.
25 Leith Court Enactment Books are in Edinburgh City Archive. Volume 1, which covers the 1680s and 90s, has details of cases, but later volumes record only the names of cautioners.
26 Unfortunately, Dundee burgh court records do not include any enactment books and did not prove usable. We made no attempt to look at Glasgow records, because the non-survival of central Glasgow kirk session registers means there would have been no way of ascertaining the relationship between ecclesiastical and civil authorities.
27 According to DesBrisay, 'Authority and Discipline', 233 and 255, in his period the burgh court dealt with criminal cases – including assault, drunkenness, theft and defamation – while civil cases came before a bailie court. Time only allowed the examination of one volume of Aberdeen court records, for the 1730s. The volume, in Aberdeen City Archive, is entitled Aberdeen Bailie Court Enactment Book and contains an extraordinarily wide range of cases: breaching the peace, theft, promises by apprentices and servants to faithfully serve their masters, commercial transactions etc. It seems likely, therefore, that the 'burgh' and 'bailie' courts were by this time combined into one. The absence of morality cases is striking.
28 DesBrisay also commented that the system survived mainly because the lack of co-operation between civil and ecclesiastical authorities earlier in the century had resulted in a lack of effective social control. 'The establishment of the justice court effectively doubled the town's capacity for social control'. Ibid., pp. 321, 368, 397.
29 Mathilda Mackie in Dundee (June 1750) said she had brought forth a child in Edinburgh but that it was 'dead born'. Although she named witnesses to the birth and burial, the session 'thought it proper that she be put in the hands of the Magistrates till she give a more particular account of the child'.
30 DesBrisay, 'Authority and Discipline', 321. Aberdeen Justice Court records are in Aberdeen City Archive.
31 When asked why she had named Mr Alexander to the session she 'answered that she had done so by bad Counsel which she professed to be sorry for & added that she had nothing to lay to Mr Alexander's Charge'.
32 Davies, 'The Courts and Scottish Legal System', p. 153.
33 That decision appears in Dundee kirk session minutes 27 December 1762.
34 Hardy, 'The Attitudes of Church and State in Scotland to Sex and Marriage', p. 471.
35 *Statistical Account of Scotland* vi (Edinburgh 1793), p. 612. Peter Vasey has brought to our notice *Ranger's Impartial List of the Ladies of Pleasure in Edinburgh*, privately published Edinburgh 1775, facsimile edition Edinburgh 1978.
36 Such cases also appear in Canongate Black Books and in Portsburgh Baron Court Book of Acts.
37 The Old Machar case was in May 1747; there were no less than five in Dundee: June 1746, April and May 1747, and two in April 1748.
38 Heinz Schilling, '"History of Crime" or "History of Sin"? Some Reflections on the Social History of Early Modern Church Discipline', in E.I. Kaurie and Tom Scott, *Politics and Society in Reformation Europe – Essays for Sir Geoffrey Elton* (London, 1987), p. 300.
39 Three weeks later the ministers advised the session that 'in their private Conversation with him he appeared neither so Ignorant nor so hardened as the Session at first had reason to apprehend', and he was allowed to satisfy. But in March 1785 he was laid under the sentence of lesser excommunication for disobedience.
40 Clark, *A History of Church Discipline*, pp. 142–3.
41 Before 1741 the timing of spontaneous confession by women was slightly later in the

pregnancy than was reporting of the pregnancy by elders: for instance, between 1711 and 1720 the average gestation of those delated was 24½ weeks, of those reporting themselves 26 weeks. After that, delation by elders became slightly later and the two figures coincide. It seems probable that a women waited until the quickening of her foetus convinced her that she was definitely pregnant and then another few weeks to summon up courage.

42 We discussed the changing ethos in *Girls in Trouble,* pp. 34–7.
43 E.g. Hugo Arnot, *Collection and Abridgement of Celebrated Criminal Trials in Scotland, 1536–1784* (Edinburgh, 1785), p. 310.
44 John, Robert and David Scotland vs. the minister of Dunfermline, 1776, W. Morison, *Dictionary of Decisions* vol. 4, pp. 9–15.

3

Control of Non-Sexual Offences

There is no denying the fact that in the eighteenth-century urban kirk sessions, in common with their counterparts in rural Scotland, appear to have been obsessed with sex, other sins being left, on the whole, to the civil courts. Of necessity, the emphasis in this book is therefore also on sexual misdemeanours, although at certain times and in certain parishes sexual cases were actually outnumbered by other kinds. Drunkenness, violence, and, above all, Sabbath breach were dealt with by kirk sessions as well as by civil courts and form the subject of this chapter.[1]

In 1672 an Act of Parliament was passed against 'profaneness', with further Acts in 1690, 1693, 1695, 1696 and 1701. Those statutes brought together previous Acts against cursing, swearing, drunkenness, and Sabbath breach. However, it was up to the church courts to refer offenders to the civil magistrates for the execution of existing laws. In 1681 a case heard by the Privy Council confirmed that the powers of civil courts to punish offenders depended on kirk sessions requesting them to do so, and at that time the Privy Council added that kirk sessions had the same powers to impose fines as justices of the peace. It seems likely that the willingness of Parliament to pass laws against profaneness after 1690 was because both the Government and the Church were newly established, and both needed the support of the other.[2] (Of course, the string of statutes can also be seen as an indication that none of them had proved effective.)

Early modern Scottish cities were full of brawling, quarrelling individuals, like Elspeth Reid in Leith who, in July 1684, was 'incarcerat within the tolbuth of the toun for scolding, flyteing with and abuseing her nyghbours contrare to christian conversation'.[3] Many such cases were instigated not by kirk sessions but by men or women complaining of others; the session's role as peacemaker should not be underestimated. (It must be remembered that there was at this time no police force, though the city guard could be called and might take brawlers into custody.)

Kirk sessions got involved not only in cases of public disturbance but also in domestic violence. For example, in Old Aberdeen in June 1674 Margaret Cumin was found guilty of 'striking and menacing hir mother'. And in Glasgow Barony in July 1701 James Adam was delated for 'abusing of his father by striking him, and giving him very irreverent language'. He 'acknowledged that he did once strike his father upon the arm'. The session 'did sharply rebuke him for this horrid & unnaturall sin', and he was ordered to be rebuked publicly.

Striking parents was unnatural; beating children, servants and wives was acceptable. Wife beating came before sessions if this happened on the Sabbath, if injury was severe enough as to incapacitate the woman, or if the uproar was such as to cause a public scandal. In August 1675 Thomas Jamesone, coachman, was cited before South Leith session for 'abuseing his wyfe in tearing her clothes & strykeing her'. He acknowledged that 'he teared the shirt off her & stroke her with his foot' and was 'therefore ordered to prison.' John Lauder appeared before the same session in February 1704 and 'confessed he was in drink and that he beat his wife & called her damned bitch and said she provocked him to it, but said it was the first tyme he had done it and hoped it would be the last. He was admonished & rebuked with certificatione that if he was seen drunk again or found to beat his wife he would be rebuked befor the congregation & referred to the Magistrats'.

In Edinburgh St Cuthbert's session (July 1712) William Steven, thatcher, was reported guilty of 'habitual drunkenness, particularly upon saturday last the 26th instant he was beastly drunk and did curse, swear and barbarously strike his wife'. When Steven appeared before the court a fortnight later, 'the session observing him to be drunk thought him incapable of Discipline Therefore they did, and hereby doe referr him to the Magistrate to incarcerate him, in order to make him more sober against the next day of his compearance.' This had the desired effect and when he was next before them he professed a 'sense of sorrow' for his behaviour '& promised through God's Strength to guard against that beastly Sin.' The session let him off with a private rebuke and the usual threat of public appearances if he was found guilty again. Unfortunately, in such a case there is no way of knowing whether he mended his ways or continued to abuse his wife in ways that did not cause scandal.

In seventeenth and eighteenth century Scotland heavy consumption of alcohol was the norm, and alcoholism was rife.[4] Just as today, when simple drunkenness is not an offence but 'drunk and disorderly' and 'drunk and incapable' are, so kirk sessions clearly ignored drunkenness up to a certain level, only taking action in cases of 'beastly drunkenness' which led to all kinds of anti-social behaviour like cursing, swearing and fighting. Such behaviour was considered particularly offensive when it happened on the Sabbath. In Edinburgh Trinity College in April 1710 a man was drunk on the Saturday night '& on the Sabbath day came out of his house naked & Danced'. In the same parish, in June 1706, Mr Roderick Mckinzie, secretary to the Africa Company, was reported 'so horridlie drunk the last Lords day in the morning, that he could neither goe nor stand Likewayes he and some others with him made such a great noise in the Back stairs in Milnes Squair... by Ranting, Singing, Curseing and Swearing which was abominable to hear, Espetiallie at such a time wherby God was greatlie dishonoured and neighbours offended by their miscarriage, which ought not to be suffered amongst Christians.'

Drinking, then as now, loosened inhibitions, and since cursing and swearing were so much frowned upon, they were an inevitable consequence. South Leith session noted in July 1702 that Margaret Brodie, apprehended by the constable, 'being excessively drunk and when she was seized upon she said – what? am I a thieff, Christ curse you all, God curse you, devill take me if I goe with you'. She was forced to endure a public rebuke for her behaviour.

Ecclesiastical historians have often claimed that the seventeenth-century Episcopal church did not have the same concern with non-sexual aspects of disorderly behaviour as the Presbyterian establishment that followed. We commented in *Girls in Trouble* that we found no real difference between the Episcopal and Presbyterian churches in this matter.[5] However, there is no denying that in the 1690s certain urban parishes, most notably South Leith and Edinburgh's West Kirk (St Cuthbert's), witnessed an enormous upsurge of zeal in prosecuting cases of cursing, swearing, 'scolding', 'scandalising' etc. This was, of course, a period of some turmoil and upheaval, with the replacement of one monarch, government and church

Sin in the City

by another. In St Cuthbert's in October 1693 Archbald Gilmoir was delated 'for drunkenness, reproach and striking his wife, and bidding damne all the whigs'. (He confessed and was ordered to appear publicly, as well as pay a civil fine.) In November 1695 Janet Craig appeared before the same session 'and declared that Doritie Corstoun cursed her and hers these three yeares... and also cursed all the presbyterians and blamed them for the badness of the weather and dearness of the meall'. Also in St Cuthbert's, in November 1707, one of the elders

> gave in a dreadfull complaint against Adam Winram bearing that the said Adam was an habitual swearer, Drunkard & moacker of religion, and particularly one time laying aside all fear of God, Did most impiously say that King William (of blessed memory) his soul was frying in hell's fire, and Devill an honest man there was in the westkirk paroch.

The civil authorities co-operated fully with the Church in attempting to put a stop to such behaviour. In March 1709 Dundee session decided to take action in regard to 'the abounding swearing & cursing amongst people in the streits' and asked the minister to speak with the magistrates 'that they would appoynt privat censurs to discover thes that swear openly on the streits & are scandalously drunk on mercat dayes that they may be openly rebuked'. The minister reported back that the magistrates promised 'to doe all they can for suppressing of vice & immoralities in this place & they shall appoynt censurs for that effect'.

During the first half of our period witchcraft was believed in, and witches were being burned in Scotland. It is beyond the scope of this book to discuss the witchcraft phenomenon, but one's expectation would be that any accusation of this 'crime' would have to be taken very seriously. The reality of kirk sessions' reactions in our cities is therefore surprising. In South Leith (August 1661) Margaret Black gave in a bill of complaint against Issobell Johnstone

> in that shee called her a witch behind her back, which the said Issobell confessit, and that she had spoken it rashlie and was sory for it, and that shee kend nothing to her but ane honest woman. Therefore the session ordained the said Issobell to sitt doune upon her knees in presence of the session, and crave Gods mercie, and the said Margarets forgiveness, which the said Issobell did willinglie and with tears, and took the said Margaret by the hand and promised never to say the lyk in tyme coming.

In the same parish in April 1664 Catheren Fairfull was referred to the civil magistrate to pay her civil penalty 'for calling Margaret Huttone witches gait, and that Margaret Black her mother may be burnt for a witch'. Catheren also had to appear publicly before the congregation for her offence. Also in Leith (November 1672) Christean Hunter, who called Margaret Shean a witch, claiming she could prove it, was referred to the civil magistrate who was to see 'hou shee would prove her a witch, other wayes to tak order with her accordinglie for scandalizing [slandering] the poor old woman as they shall judge expedient.' Margaret Nisbet complainer and Marion Dunlop defender appeared before Edinburgh St Cuthbert's session in August 1704. The defender, Marion, confessed that she had called Margaret a witch, because 'her child being unwell [she] gott a drink of some herbs from the said Margaret and after he had a little received the same, he died, and thereby she judged that Margaret was the Devill's servant'. The moderator 'most smartly rebuked the said Marion for her

3: Control of Non-Sexual Offences

horrid wickedness in slandering her neighbour and ordered her to live more peaceablie in time comeing which she promised to doe, & in token of reconcilement he enjoyned them to mutual shakeing of hands, which was done accordinglie, and the session referred the said Marion to the Magistrat to bind her to the peace with the said Margaret and her familie.'

We found no examples of an accusation of witchcraft being believed or acted upon. As is clear from Christina Larner's work, there had to be specific circumstances in a particular locality for witchcraft hysteria to blow up.[6] When a minister was well acquainted with a woman so accused he was in a position to dismiss the notion that there might be any truth in it.

The offence that preoccupied sessions above all was Sabbath breach. The Bible enjoined a day of rest, but it took the Reformation Church to turn this into a day when nothing but church services and religious study were to be allowed. The basic human needs of rest and recreation were not to be indulged. In April 1667 Canongate session recommended that elders and deacons look out for children playing after the afternoon's sermon and give their names to the session, 'and that schoolmasters and schoolmistresses tak their schollers to the schoole upon the lords day and tak accompt of them what they have heard of the sermons'. However, as with other types of non-sexual offences, the replacement of the Episcopal church by a Presbyterian establishment in the 1690s saw a terrific upsurge in cases of Sabbath breach.

During this period many sessions instigated a system of 'searchers': members of session who would take it in turn to patrol the streets during services and delate anyone who was not in church to the next session meeting. Some members of Dundee session complained in August 1703 that although ale house keepers would give them access 'yet they will not allow them to search some particular rooms in the houss'; in consequence the session passed an act that anyone refusing access to any room would be referred to the bailie for civil punishment and rebuked sessionally for a first fault and publicly for a second. In both St Cuthbert's and South Leith in the late 1690s and early 1700s, cases of Sabbath breach far outnumbered cases of fornication and adultery. (But treatment of offenders was different: a first Sabbath breach offence led only to a rebuke in front of the session, whereas any sexual offence required a rebuke in front of the congregation.)

In spite of the Church's strictures, some people continued to regard the Sabbath as a day of rest and enjoyment. 'Vaiging' or 'idly walking' crops up constantly in parishes throughout Scotland. Sometimes individuals were cited, but more often public intimation was made from the pulpit because the numbers involved were too large for individuals to be singled out. 'Vaiging' was considered an offence even if folk had been to church, as is clear from a complaint made by Dundee session in January 1704 of 'people walking in the fields after Sermon & on the shoar at night'. Fourteen years later, in May 1718, the session was still unhappy about 'people walking on the shoar and in the fields before and after sermon'.

In St Cuthbert's parish in August 1721 a man and his wife were reported for being idle on the Sabbath, the man having been found in his bed 'tho' in perfite health'. The woman appeared before the session (her husband being away on business) and admitted that they had both been at home the previous Sabbath, 'but were doing no harm, for her Husband was lying in his bed reading upon a book & she keeping their young child'. Such a response seems entirely reasonable to the modern reader, but the session clerk recorded that she 'was in no way sensible of any fault she had done, being quite Ignorant that the Lord's day is prophaned by idleness.'

That particular session had to contend not only with its own parishioners but with many city centre parishioners as well, who clearly enjoyed breathing in the fresh air of the surrounding countryside. An offence which cropped up regularly in the parish in the early eighteenth century was swimming. The first mention of this occurs in July 1710 when three young men were rebuked for 'swimming in Bonningtoun Water'. The numbers engaging in this pastime increased in the years that followed, so that by July 1718 the session referred to 'multitudes of people idly walking in the fields and bathing themselves in the water'.

Because of this the session recommended that the moderator write to the lord provost of Edinburgh 'in order to procure an order from his Lordship for a competent number of soldiers in the city-guard to attend upon the Elders and Diacons every Lord's day that they goe to Boningtoun water for suppressing effectually these horrid Outrages on the Lord's day.' The moderator reported to the session that no sooner did the lord provost receive his letter than he sent orders to the Captain of the city guard and advised the session 'that he would not only send soldiers to Boningtoun, but any where else of the parioch under the Jurisdiction of the City where the Lord's day was prophaned.' This is a good illustration of the way in which the civil authorities concurred with the kirk's view of morality, and of their willingness to assist in controlling behaviour that was considered unchristian. But the offence continued, and in May 1723 the assistance of soldiers was again being sought, 'to suppress swimming in Boningtoun water on the Lord's day, it being scandalous to see such swarms of people resort there on the said day for that End.' A similar request for assistance was made in May 1733 and again in 1738.[7]

That particular behaviour was unique to the West Kirk parish, but one offence could be found in every urban parish in the land: entertaining people on the Sabbath. Having the odd drink after services might be acceptable, but plying folk with drink instead of being in church was not, and it was offenders of this kind who were the main target of the 'searchers' when they perambulated the streets. There were no licensing laws at the time, but it is noteworthy that usually only those doing the entertaining were rebuked; presumably those being entertained belonged to other parishes.

Not all Sabbath breakers were being self-indulgent, for carrying out workday tasks was as much a fault. Work was only permitted if it could be proven to be 'of necessity'. In Dundee in October 1707 two boatmen were cited for ferrying passengers. They declared that some gentlemen 'would not be denyed passage'. The session clearly appreciated the difficulty in saying no to gentry but required the boatmen to 'shun all temptations of that nature as much as they can'. In January 1708 the catechist gave in a list of names of ferrymen whom he saw in boats when he was going to Monifieth to preach. They declared 'it was but to cast their Boats dry on the Sab: least they should sink in the river they lookt upon that as a work of necessitie'. The session accepted that this was genuine necessity, while the ferrymen promised 'to observe the Lord's day better'. It is amazing to think of sessions taking so much trouble to investigate such things, but it indicates their strength of feeling on the matter.

In the 1690s the session of St Cuthbert's parish on the outskirts of Edinburgh dealt with many cases of people bringing milk into the city. To give some examples: in December 1697 a man was cited because his family was 'carrieing in great Stoups full of milk in to Edr'. He claimed not to know that his family or servants did this. His wife admitted sending milk to the city, 'but it was in Litle Stoups, it's true her servant had a big Stoup in her hand but she had it not in Edr, she only brought it out of her neighbour's house'. But the servant admitted guilt, and she and her master were rebuked. In April 1698 a man who confessed 'sending out his servetrix to sell milk in great stoups on the Sabbath days & of keeping mercats thereof' had to appear before the congregation for this offence.

The practice continued in the following decade. In January 1705 intimation was made from the pulpit 'discharging [prohibiting] milk to be carried in the city in such great quantities on the Lord's day'. It was obviously considered futile to forbid all carrying and selling of milk, and at the end of the decade the session, fulminating against 'the habitual scandalous prophanation of the Lord's day, by carrying of Milk to the City in great Quantities, notwithstanding of the many former essays they have made for suppressing of that Scandall', recommended that the magistrates take measures. They were to forbid all those who sold milk on the Sabbath to carry in more than a quart at one time, and to be restricted to doing so before seven in the morning in summer and eight in the morning in winter. This compromise appears to have worked, or else the session simply gave up, for there is no further mention of the offence in later decades.

It was not at all unusual for sinners caught by the 'searchers' to become verbally, and sometimes even physically, abusive at the time (which naturally exacerbated the initial offence in the session's eyes), but they nearly always appeared before the session when cited and apologised for their behaviour. But what about the gentry? In September 1705 report was made to St Cuthbert's session of an 'unparalleled prophanation of the Lord's day', and from the details which followed that description was not exaggerated. Four gentlemen – Hugh Shaw, brother to the Laird of Greenock, William Graham, son to the Laird of Douglastoun, Robert Rae, son to Lieutenant Colonel Rae, and John Harbertsone of Barachnie – went drinking and after some 'prophane singing and danceing' they

> attempted to commit a rape upon one or two women; Did with their swords wound to the effusion of blood several women & one man, Did use most horrid curseing imprecations threaten the murder of one man & some women... And did with their hands & feet beat & hurt a great many women, Did break several glass-windows with stones, Did throw in great stones upon a woman lying in child-bed, so that it was a wonder that both she and her child were not murdered, and so desperate & brutal was their madness, that they fell upon even such beasts as fell in their way, Insomuch as they killed with their swords a Greyhound outright, pierced another Dog through the bellie, and threw stones at, and either killed or hurt several Cocks and hens.

It seems extraordinary that the session register makes no mention of any criminal proceedings initiated against them, but they appeared before the presbytery, and in January 1706 they made a public appearance in front of the congregation where they were 'gravely and smartly rebuked' by the minister; the gentlemen 'behaved very gravely, and professed a sense of their horrid provocations in face of the Congregation.' It may say something about the strength of church discipline in this period that they all conformed, or perhaps they were threatened with more severe civil punishment if they did not do so?

Sin in the City

In March 1724 South Leith session was informed that 'some Gentlemen were playing at the Golf in the Links of Leith on Sabbath last'. The men – named as Gourlay of Kincraig, Moncrieff of Reedy, '& a son of Captain Cramonds' – had apparently got clubs from John Dickson, 'golf club maker', who with his wife had afterwards entertained them, while a young lad, James Aiken, 'was employed in carrying their clubs'. Not content with rebuking Dickson and his spouse 'for entertaining people whom they knew to be guilty of such enormities on the Lords day', and the lad, the session were determined to get at the gentlemen as well. Two of them appeared shortly afterwards; 'both confessed their great fault & heinous offence, & professed great sorrow & shame for the same.' They promised to appear again whenever called and meanwhile the session referred the case to presbytery.

The presbytery, having 'discoursed at great length' on this, 'Did judge the open playing at the Golf on the publick Links of Leith upon the Lords day, or going about with Players, to be an Heinous profanation of that Holy day', so much so that the sentence of lesser excommunication might be passed against them. However, as they had voluntarily appeared and confessed their fault, the presbytery advised that the gentlemen should simply appear before the congregation and be publicly rebuked. The session subsequently spent years trying to get them to make their appearances, but without success. As will be discussed in a later chapter, this was all too often the case with gentry, and the main point here is the Church's strength of feeling against such activity on the Sabbath.

In view of this, the question is why Sabbath breach cases subsequently disappear from kirk session registers. Stephen Davies wrote that Justice of the Peace courts expanded their range of business after 1707 to include punishing Sabbath breakers, which 'accounts for the decline in the number of such cases processed by the church courts after 1708.'[8] 'Crimes' like cursing and swearing certainly appear in the Edinburgh JP court records, as in the case of Anne Dale, who in November 1736 complained that when her husband was absent Alison Cheap would call her 'whore, strumpet, Limmer, Bitch, Street whore, that she Lay in the Street with a man & many other ill names And was also accustomed to Imprecate that the Devill might turn the Complainer inside out and putt her in hell And that God might damn and sink her to Eternity'.[9] However, the minutes of that court contain no Sabbath breach cases whatsoever. Nor is there any dramatic dropping off of Sabbath breach cases in kirk session registers at such an early date. We must therefore look elsewhere for an explanation.

There are two possible assumptions that one could make. The first is that the concept of Sabbath as a holy day (or at the very least, of a day when one could not be seen to be doing anything) became so internalised that there were no offenders for sessions to rebuke. The second is that sessions gave up worrying about Sabbath breach, choosing to concentrate solely on sexual misdemeanours.

The first of these receives strong support from the records of sessions which continued to employ 'searchers', South Leith being the most consistent. Between 1711 and 1720 Sabbath breakers were reported nearly every week, and sometimes a woman's plaid (on one occasion a 'pint stoup') was taken to ensure her appearance. From 1721 to 1730 the 'searchers' were as assiduous as ever, and Sabbath breakers were still appearing before the session. By the 1730s 'searching' still went on, but more often than not there was nothing to report. In the 1740s weekly searchers continued to be carried out, but in the whole decade only a handful of Sabbath breakers were actually found.

What about other parishes? In Glasgow Barony a case in December 1741 illustrates that parishioners and the session still took Sabbath breach very seriously. The moderator reported that John Wilson had admitted working one harvest-time Sabbath 'among his bear [barley]' and had alleged it was necessary because 'thro a whole week of heavy rains it was in the outmost danger of perishing'. When he appeared before the session he was asked 'what he had done among his Victuall some Sabbath in Harvest last, at which the Neighbourhood was so much offended'. He still claimed that 'he thought it Incumbent on him to get up the sheaves and carry the Victual from a low moist place where it was standing to a higher ground'. He said that 'had he known it would have given so much offence he would not have done it, and promis'd to do so no more', but this was not enough for the session. They all felt that 'there could be no Necessity for such a practice last Harvest which was extreamly favourable' and that he would have to admit his fault and express sorrow for it. When he was called back in he did so and was rebuked for the sin.

In Canongate in the 1740s there were a number of cases of cursing, swearing and drunkenness, but only two of Sabbath breach. In October 1748 two women were found guilty of carrying buckets of water through the streets and sessionally rebuked. In August 1749 a man who had already been found guilty of cursing and swearing, profaned the Sabbath by taking boys out to climb trees; he also threw stones at windows and broke some of them. The session 'considering all this... were of opinion that they would concern themselves no more with such a Wicked Villain; and applied to the magistrates 'that he be banished the Toun'. But, rather surprisingly, in May 1747 the town council actually asked that elders and deacons join with the constables to walk the streets during sermons 'and apprehend every disorderly person'.

The notion that Sabbath breach had entirely disappeared by then gains even less credence when one discovers that Edinburgh presbytery produced an act specifically against this offence in June 1740, prohibiting 'not only such works as are at all times Sinful' but also 'all worldly Employment and business, Diversions and recreations as are lawfull on other days', and stressing 'faithful performance of the duties of public prayers and sacred worship', 'except as much of the day as is to be taken upon the Works of necessitie and mercy'.

Some parishioners began to question the need for this. For example, in August 1743 William Sangster, mason in Aberdeen, was asked why he allowed his children 'to entertain their Comrades and Strangers in his Garden on the Sabbath day'. He replied that he 'thought there is no fault in so doing, and said they might be as well there as elsewhere, and behav'd himself insolently to the Session'. (The session referred him to the magistrates 'to be punish'd as Law allows and bound to the observation of the Lord's day'.) In North Leith in April 1754 various individuals were cited for carrying water and kale on the Sabbath, expressed repentance and were dismissed, but John Sherriff 'said he thought it was no fault nor breach of the Sabbath to carry or cause carry Kail or Water if he needed them; And when the Moderator endeavoured to convince him that such practises were really a breach of the Sabbath, he impudently said they were not; And that for his part he would carry home what his Family needed, and let the session do their best.' (He too was referred to the civil magistrate.)

In April 1750 Aberdeen session was advised that the presbytery intended to

Sin in the City

prosecute several salmon fishers who went fishing on the Sabbath, 'before the Civil as well as the Ecclesiastic courts'. The presbytery desired the concurrence of the session 'in contributing to defray the expence of a Prosecution'. The session agreed to do so and also appointed a committee 'to wait upon the Honourable the Magistrates and represent to them the great abuse and profanation of the Lord's day, and to desire their Concurrence and Assistance in suppressing the same.' In response the magistrates 'emitted a proclamation by tuck of Drum against that practice.'

The fact that individuals did not appear before kirk sessions for Sabbath breach in the later decades of the eighteenth century does not mean that such breaches were ignored. It was reported to Aberdeen session in June 1764 that the Lord's day 'was greatly profaned by carrying in water in Buckets, and walking in the streets and fields.' The magistrates were asked to 'interpose their authority to prevent the like practice in all time coming.' Three years later, in August 1767, it was observed that 'the sabbath is at present violated in the most open manner in this place'; once again recourse was had to the magistrates.

In May 1784 a complaint was made to that session that a military band had been playing during the past few Sabbaths, 'by which means a large unruly Mob of idle people are gathered together, and many Indecencies & abuses committed'. The session spelled out in more detail their objections to 'such Musical Meetings at any time upon the Lords day': they were 'very offensive to the sincere & pious of all denominations, and tending to promote a Spirit of Dissipation among the young, the thoughtless, and the giddy, teaching them to despise the Sabbath day & thus corrupting their morals & leading them into many dangerous fatal snares.' The session applied to the magistrates, 'entreating that they will exert their Authority in putting a stop to such practices in all time coming'. The lord provost assured the session that everything possible would be done to accomplish this end.

Not all kirk sessions had recourse to civil authorities for this offence. When Dundee considered a gross abuse of the Sabbath in November 1778, 'by several of the Inhabitants of this place by the driving of Cloth on the streets and shiping of the [cloth] on Board of James Browns Vessel', they decided that 'all such as had been concerned in that matter & are in Communion with the Church of Scotland should be censured'. In November 1782

> The Session considering that the profanation of the Lords Day was becoming customary in this place by Persons frequenting public Houses on the Lords Day and drinking there after Divine Service were of opinion that a Stop should be put this prevailing custom – They therefore agree that if any of those Persons who keep public Houses & belong to the established Church shall allow any person or persons to frequent their Houses on the Lords Day & sell them Drink of any kind, unless in case of Necessity shall be cut off from Church Privileges & that the same Sentence should be execute against those persons who frequent said Houses.

Twelve years later, in August 1794, that session, 'having with regret taken into their serious consideration how much the Lords day hath of late been and still is profaned by many persons in various ways, and particularly by bathing in the sea; unanimously agreed that such a public & gross breach of the sabbath should be prohibited for the future from the Pulpits'. They also agreed that if the practice continued, 'application shall be made to the Magistrates to have the law executed upon the offenders according to an Act of Parliament.' So, in the end, even Dundee had to utilise the civil authorities.

Nevertheless, it would be incorrect to claim that Sabbath breach continued as prevalent as it had been earlier in the century, and that kirk sessions simply sloughed the problem onto the civil magistrates. To a greater or lesser extent, the idea of the sanctity of the Lord's day did become internalised during the course of our period. Indeed, it continued to gain strength in the nineteenth century and through much of the twentieth, though more so in rural Scotland than in cities.

However, at the same time as this was happening the monolithic church structure was breaking down, and once individuals had a choice of belonging or not belonging to the established church, the Church's control over parishioners' activities on a Sunday was broken. It is clear that civil authorities were in complete sympathy with kirk sessions over this issue in all the Scottish cities, but their chances of putting a complete stop to Sunday activity became increasingly remote.

Notes

Edinburgh, Canongate and Leith kirk session registers are in the Scottish Record Office; the only exception is Edinburgh New Kirk which for the year 1706 is in Edinburgh University Library and for several other years in Edinburgh City Archive. Aberdeen St Nicholas registers are in Aberdeen City Archive; Old Machar registers are in the parish church, with access via Aberdeen University – microfilms of both sessions' records are in the Scottish Record Office. Glasgow Barony and Govan session registers are in Glasgow City Archive, and have not been microfilmed. Dundee registers are in Dundee City Archive, with microfilms in Edinburgh. We have not given references for each citation but always state the month and year, making it possible for anyone to find a particular case.

1. Some of the material in this chapter formed part of a paper entitled 'The kirk session and social control in early-modern Scottish cities – a preliminary enquiry', delivered by Leah Leneman at the ASHS conference, St Andrews, October 1993. See also Leah Leneman, '"Prophaning" the Lord's Day – Sabbath Breach in Early Modern Scotland', *History,* Vol. 241 (1989).
2. J.R. Hardy, 'The Attitudes of Church and State in Scotland to Sex and Marriage, 1500–1707' (unpublished M.Phil. thesis, University of Edinburgh, 1978), pp. 444–5, 451.
3. Leith Court Enactment Books Vol. 1, Edinburgh City Archive.
4. Our comment on alcoholism being rife comes from Leah Leneman's research on divorce based on consistory court records, where it is clear that this was often a cause of marital breakdown.
5. *Girls in Trouble: Sexuality and Social Control in Rural Scotland 1660–1780* (Edinburgh, 1998), p. 11.
6. Christina Larner, *Enemies of God* (London, 1981).
7. Was there perhaps considered to be an element of indecency in young people larking about in the water without many clothes on? This is never mentioned, though it is not impossible.
8. Stephen J. Davies, 'The Courts and the Scottish Legal System 1600–1747: The Case of Stirlingshire', in V.C. Gatrell, Bruce Lenman and Geoffrey Parker (eds.), *Crime and the Law* (London, 1980), p. 134.
9. SRO.JP35/4/2.

4

The Background to Illegitimacy and Bridal Pregnancy

Before grappling with the quantitative evidence for illegitimacy in our cities there is a great deal to be learned from kirk session records about the behaviour that led to our statistics. One fundamental difference between urban and rural parishes is that most illegitimate children born in a rural parish were conceived there, which is by no means the case for city parishes. Women bearing bastards would come to Edinburgh in the hope of losing themselves in the anonymity of the city, sometimes leaving the infant behind.

In Trinity College parish (September 1702) Alison Whyt was 'found upon the streets likely to bring forth ane chyld'. She was taken to the constable's house where she gave birth, and was then sent back to her home parish. Jane Davidson appeared before Edinburgh St Cuthbert's session (June 1711) and said that she had been guilty with Charles Longreach in Aberdeen. 'And declared that the said Charles advised her to goe to Edinr when she was 20 weeks gone, and she came to the house of one Robert Cuming coach-man in the Canongate, where also she was brought to bed, and gave a shilling to an Episcopal Incumbent to baptize her child'. She was ordered to find a cautioner that she would appear before Aberdeen session.

Dundee session dealt with such cases from time to time, but women there did not always comply with their partner's wishes. Barbara Gib (August 1731) named John Wedderburn, son of Bailie Wedderburn, as father of her child, and said she had told him she was pregnant, 'and he desired her to goe to Edr and bear the child which she refused to doe'. Elizabeth Lawson (August 1766) said that her partner admitted paternity in front of her master and mistress, 'and proposed in their hearing that she should leave this Town, go to Edinburgh and bear her Child, and that he would bear her Expences.' In June 1737 Isobel Wilson denied having gone to Edinburgh to bear an illegitimate child. She said that she had gone away because 'she hade disobliged her Father in staying with My Lady Sinclar' – connections which reveal she was of the gentry class – and that she had stayed with her brother in Leith. By August the session had located a witness who declared that Isobel 'was confined three days in Alexr Swines Kirk Trsr his mans house att Edr and that she brought forth a child in a Taylors house in Cowlls Closs and that she hade the child in her Arms two hours and that Provost Ramsays Daughter went very near her and that the child was called Geills after Provost Ramsays Daughter and that the child was Gleid [squint-eyed]'. Isobel confessed that the child was born the previous August, 'baptised by ane Episcopal Minister', and was still alive. By the end of our period Dundee was a big enough city for women to come from outlying rural areas to bear their illegitimate children there. Jean White (July 1779), 'being asked from whence she had come replied that she came from Forgandenny… being asked for what Intent she had come

4: The Background to Illegitimacy and Bridal Pregnancy

to this Place replied that she was with Child to John Rutherford in Perth & that she had left her People on Account of their looking down upon her'. Dundee session had scant sympathy; they 'recommended it to her to return home again with all convenient speed otherwise Application would be made to a Magistrate to have her put away publicly'.

City sessions naturally did all they could to try and stop women coming to their parishes to be delivered of unwanted children. The system of requiring a testimonial from anyone entering a parish was supposed to serve that purpose, but women coming to a city to give birth often had partners who could pay for lodgings. In December 1699 South Leith session were angry at Mistress Scott because a woman from another parish had a child in her house: 'The Session considering that the Magistrats had made ane Act discharging [prohibiting] all hous keepers to take in any strangers to their houses for any considerable tyme without sufficient testimonialls under the pain of twentie pound Scots, And had caused intimat the samen through the toun by touck of Drum, They doe reffer to the magistrats to cause put the same in executione against Mistress Scott'.

One group whom urban sessions attempted to use in their efforts at control were midwives, since they would be called upon by all women bearing children, whether belonging to the parish or not. For this reason Edinburgh made all midwives sign a bond declaring that they would report the names of any stranger women they assisted.[1] The West Kirk parish session (St Cuthbert's) drew up its own bond in December 1718 and reproduced the text in their minutes; this appears as Appendix 1. Meanwhile, in May 1715 South Leith session summoned all of the midwives in their parish: 'Being enquired if they had brought any stranger woman to bed, within these two monethe, they said all, none. They were discharged in time comeing to assist any stranger in Child birth, till first they acquaint some of the members of Session thereof, or att least immediately thereafter with certification if the Contrary they would be referred to the Magistrats for so doing'.

We cannot know how effective the bond was, but there were certainly slip-ups. In April 1724 a midwife was cited before New Greyfriars session for assisting Mary Livingston, who had subsequently fled. She declared that Mary's landlord and landlady told her 'that the said Mary was Married and that her husband was at Sea, which she the declarant believed, and therefore did perform the office of a Midwife to her. The Modr gravely & sharply rebuked her for not acquainting the Magistrats or session anent the said Mary she knowing her to be a stranger & she being enjoined if afterward she should be called to bring any such person to bed that she would give timeous advertisement thereof'.

In September 1749 Aberdeen session only discovered that Anne Knox had borne a child more than a year after she had done so and chased up the midwife who had assisted her. After admitting that 'she had neglected to inform the Magistrates or Ministers of her having so done', she was rebuked, 'and strictly enjoin'd to acquaint both the magistrates and the Ministers in the like case in all time coming'. Again, we cannot know how often midwives did collude with women to keep an illegitimate birth secret.

Sessions learned about unmarried women being pregnant through local gossip. A conscientious session was likely to detect more women at an early stage of pregnancy than a more lax session. The stage of pregnancy at which women were cited cannot be ascertained for all our parishes, but over several decades South Leith,

Sin in the City

North Leith, Aberdeen, and Dundee sessions routinely asked women when their child was conceived. We divided terms into 'under 5 months', '5 to 8 months', '9th month', and 'child born'. Not surprisingly, in all the above parishes, in most decades, the majority of women were between five and eight months pregnant when they were cited. But there were differences between parishes and over time.

As Tables 4.1 and 4.2 reveal, in the decade between 1711 and 1720 South Leith and Aberdeen followed roughly similar patterns, with about a quarter of women being cited after their illegitimate child was born, and the great majority being cited long before that. Aberdeen clearly lost its grip to some extent in the 1720s but regained it in the 1730s. The shift in the 1740s, when approximately half the citations were of women who had already borne their children, or were just about to do so, is striking. The information is not given for any later period, but it seems likely that the percentage would have paralleled South Leith's, where some 62 per cent of women fell into that category, and no pregnancy was discovered under five months.

Table 4.1: Months pregnant when discovered by session: South Leith
(not including self-delations and referrals from other parishes)

	0–5 Months (%)	5–8 Months (%)	8–9 Months (%)	Child born (%)	Total sample
1711–20	8 (15)	32 (61)	5 (10)	8 (15)	52
1721–30	5 (9)	29 (54)	5 (9)	15 (28)	54
1731–40	7 (14)	22 (43)	3 (6)	19 (37)	51
1741–50	0 (0)	17 (51)	2 (6)	14 (42)	33
1751–60	0 (0)	9 (37)	2 (8)	13 (54)	24

Table 4.2: Months pregnant when discovered by session: Aberdeen St Nicholas

	0–5 Months (%)	5–8 Months (%)	8–9 Months (%)	Child born (%)	Total sample
1711–20	10 (11)	62 (67)	8 (9)	12 (13)	92
1721–30	5 (13)	16 (43)	5 (13)	11 (30)	37
1731–40	11 (16)	43 (61)	7 (10)	9 (13)	70
1741–50	5 (8)	25 (40)	8 (13)	23 (38)	61

Dundee's pattern, as shown in Table 4.3, was very different. As late as the 1740s only about 22 per cent of women were caught after, or just before, the birth of the child. Though by the 1770s the percentage had risen to some 31 per cent – still very much lower than Aberdeen or South Leith in earlier decades – 13 per cent were caught under five months, which was as high a percentage as most sessions had managed much earlier in the century.[2]

4: The Background to Illegitimacy and Bridal Pregnancy

Table 4.3: Months pregnant when discovered by session: Dundee

	0–5 Months (%)	5–8 Months (%)	8–9 Months (%)	Child born (%)	Total sample
1731–40	7 (13)	22 (43)	3 (6)	19 (37)	51
1741–50	9 (29)	17 (51)	2 (6)	14 (42)	33
1751–60	\multicolumn{4}{Not enough information}	
1761–70	11 (17)	34 (51)	2 (3)	19 (29)	66
1771–80	16 (13)	65 (54)	8 (7)	32 (26)	121

Urban women were more likely to deny being pregnant than their rural counterparts. In Aberdeen Jean Robertson denied being pregnant at the beginning of December, saying that she 'had been in a bad state of health for about two years and a half preceding. The session recommended it to her mother who is here present to keep a strict Eye over her till Whitsunday next and to report to the session if she proves with child'. In the event, there was no need to wait until Whitsunday, for her child was born in March.

Catherine Cameron's denial to Glasgow Barony session was even more audacious. On 7 July 1765

> she absolutely refused that she is with Child, But acknowledged that she had a mind to have gone home to the Highlands to see her friends But that upon the breaking out of that report anent her, she had altered her Resolution and resolved rather to stay and make the Contrary appear. The Session not perceiving very apparent signs of pregnancy about her by her Bulk in their eyes Thought proper to defer any further enquiry anent her till time should bring the truth to light one way or other as she was to stay in the Bounds.

But she did not stay 'in the Bounds': on 14 July she had her child 'upon the highway as she was travelling towards the Highlands with a design as it is thought to have concealed the scandal here'. However, the record for a late denial must be held by Marian Dun in South Leith (December 1712): 'when she was in her pangs she denyed she was with child, and continued in her denyell till the child was heared weep'.

Usually if a woman was suspected of being with child and denied it, a midwife would be called upon to examine her. In May 1743 when Dundee session asked Christian Hay if she was with child, 'she Judicially declared with great and solemn Imprecations she was not and that it was out of malice she was brought before the Session'. Two midwives examined her and declared that she was six months gone with child. Another Dundee woman, Jean Milln (September 1771), refused to submit to an examination by a midwife after she denied being pregnant. The session applied to the provost to have her imprisoned until she submitted, 'Which having been done & she imprisoned & examined was found to be going on to six months with child'. Ultimately, a woman had no choice over submitting to such an examination.

In at least one case an examination did not reveal the truth. Margaret Brown was delated to Dundee session on 29 August 1709. On 12 September 'James Zeamen present bailie declared befor the Session that it was a meer calumnie in saying that his servant Margaret Brown was with chyld', for he had called 'his own wyff &

Sin in the City

severall other women & made them tak inspection of her breasts & the women declared that the poor Lass was mightily wronged & that she was not with chyld'. She gave birth about seven and a half months after this, so she must have been in the earliest stages of pregnancy when the report was first circulated.

However, a session could get it wrong. In Aberdeen it was reported in October 1747 that Isobel Sievewright had been delated several weeks earlier to the session as being with child in fornication; she had refused to attend the session and denied the charge so magistrates had ordered her to be examined by midwives. The midwives, 'having declared upon oath that the said Isobel Sievewright is not presently with Child, nor has brought forth one lately, the Session appointed the whole affair to be cancelled out of their Minutes'. But Isobel and her relatives were not satisfied with that and complained to the presbytery about 'the Injury done to her Character by a prosecution of this nature', so intimation was to be made 'from both pulpits, that after the strictest enquiry which the session and the Magistrates could make in the affair, the said Isobel Sievewright was found innocent.' Furthermore, it appeared that a fellow servant of hers, Robert Paterson, had played a considerable part in spreading the slander. Paterson was therefore cited before the session. He declared that he had told the neighbourhood 'what he thought to be true... namely that he suspected that the said Isobel Sievewright had really brought forth a Child some days before, and that he thought his suspicion pretty well founded'. The session rebuked him 'for his precipitancy and rashness in this matter' and admonished him 'to be more cautious of people's Characters in time coming.'[3]

An illegitimate child was usually an unwanted child, and urban women were far more likely than rural women to resort to materials believed to be abortifacients. In April 1708 Margaret Shaw told South Leith session that when she advised her partner 'that she was with child to him, he bad her take a drink as other women did to put back the child'.

In Edinburgh St Cuthbert's (January 1706) Janet Simpson, servetrix to John Watson, barber, confessed to fornication with his apprentice, David Ranny. She added that 'David gave her a powder to take among some ale, but ere she would doe it, she took the advice of some neighbours, who diswaded her from it; and told that the powder is still in her Masters Custody'. The powder was subsequently produced and retained by the session. Ranny fled the parish but returned four years later, and in April 1710 he admitted that he 'gott the powder of Joulop in an Apothercarys shop'. The session now asked a 'skillful Chirugeon' to analyse it, and he reported that 'it was the powder of Julop, and declared that David could not have given her a worse thing, for there was as much of it in a dose, as would have killed a horse.' The moderator asked David 'who advised him to buy, and where he gott such a dangerous powder? he answered he heard his master John Watson say, when Janet fell with child, if he would give her a penny worth of the Powder of Julop it would make her part with Child, and God forgive him his heart was so inclin'd, and he accordinglie went to Mistres Hair her shop'.

In July 1712 Marion Faries confessed to South Leith session that 'about ten weeks after their being guilty together she drank of Herbs and took a Vomiter'. Most of the substances considered abortifacients were aimed at producing vomiting and diarrhoea, in the vain hope that the foetus would also be expelled. Another expedient was to draw blood; the logic behind this is not known, but it is referred to so often, usually in conjunction with other methods, that there must have been a strong belief

4: The Background to Illegitimacy and Bridal Pregnancy

in its efficacy. Herbs specifically named were 'centery' and savine. Margaret Low told South Leith session in May 1712 that her partner 'gave her snuff amongst ale to make her part with child'. Jane Fairries advised St Cuthbert's session in August 1736 that James White, gardener, 'was so perverse as to gather herbs for her drink of when steeped in ale in order to put the child back, and owned that the first time she drank of the herbs she felt no harm, but when she drank it thereafter, she fell very sick, and would never again drink of it'.

When the evidence of a man's procuring herbs or 'powder' was too strong for him to deny it, the usual story was that he had done so because the woman was feeling unwell, not having realised she was carrying a child. An even more far-fetched version of this was heard by St Cuthbert's. In October 1730 Grizel Eliot declared that Robert Gray had said to her after their guilt together, 'if she found herself with child, he proposed to gett some herbs and powders... to cause abortion but she refused to take them'. Gray averred to the session that 'he understood that she was smitten with the Clap... and that made him propose to her to gett the herbs & powders to cure her'.[4]

If effective abortifacients had been readily available, there would have been far fewer illegitimate births; most such cases came to light either because the woman had refused to take anything and the man was denying paternity, or because they had not worked. However, there was at least one case where they were thought to have worked. Janet Clark, late servant and housekeeper to George Cramond, brewer, told Dundee session (November 1782) that after she realised she was with child to her master obtained 'eight papers full of herbs' from Dr Dooly: 'That Cramond took one of the papers, & steeped the herbs (in a Teapot with some warm water) and that she was ordered to steep as much each Day, & to drink the Infusion, at three different Times, the same Dose being duly repeated. That Cramond was always present when she drank this Liquor & held the Tankard to her. That she declared her Aversion to drink these Draughts both to Dr Dooly & G Cramond.' One morning, after she had taken the infusion of four of the papers, the wife of a neighbour came in one morning and saw her steeping them. She asked to see the herbs, 'and said there was Saving Tree [savine] among them' and forbade her to take any more of them, telling Cramond 'what he did was very wrong'. But after that he gave her more powders and

> on Wednesday night last week, when nobody was in the house but themselves two, He the said George Cramond took her the Declarant by the hair, and pulled her back over a Chair, & having first put a little white powder into aleberry, he forced the same into her mouth with his own hands and held her till she swallowed it, That this had a violent Effect upon her, so that she got no rest that night after but was extremely ill.

Finally she said that 'she thought herself to have been with Child, & that she parted with it by the said Drugs'. (Of course, it might have been a natural miscarriage.)

In another Dundee case (February 1790) Agnes Alison said that Ninian Alexander 'caused her to use means to provoke an abortion viz. He caused her to swallow Seventeen Mercury Pills – & made her take many a Draught of things out of Bottles (some of which she produced) which always kept her in pain till she threw them up again'. Ninian of course denied, and the doctor insisted that all he had supplied was 'a Box of Cathartic or purging pills... [and] a Bottle to the same purpose but neither of them injurious so as to do hurt to an Embryo or Foetus.' But a witness declared that Ninian told him that if Agnes was with child 'she would not bring forth a living one from which he understood that means had been used for the hurt of the child'. In the same parish three years later (February 1793) Marjory Thoms said that James Ross put something in her gin, and also in her oatmeal, and then departed, 'when she fell a throwing up & was bad for some Days'. When he returned 'she asked what it was that he put amongst her meal & the gin which made her throw up to which he answered that it was good for her that she threw up'.

Most attempted abortions appear to have been instigated by the male partner, but not always. In May 1780 James Boyd was asked 'if he had any hand in applying to one David Mitchell for medicines to Elizabeth Sharp in order to procure an abortion of her last child'. He denied having done so. Elizabeth, being asked what she wanted with Mitchell, 'answered that she did wish to get free of her last Child & wished to have Medicines for that purpose but that what ever hand James Boyd had in it was entirely owing to her'. (But he admitted paying for the 'medicines'.)

We found no references to abortions by means of 'knitting needles' or the insertion of any other devices. Whether such methods were unknown or simply considered too dangerous to attempt we cannot tell, but with accusations of all kinds flying about during kirk session appearances, we find it inconceivable that such means could have been used without ever being mentioned, or even hinted at.

Earlier in the chapter we mentioned that women often came to Edinburgh from elsewhere in Scotland to give birth to an illegitimate child. Some left that child behind. In June 1720 Janet Dalgardine confessed to Aberdeen Justice Court that two and a half years earlier she had been with child to a soldier, had gone to Edinburgh where 'she brought furth a female child, and about eight or ten dayes after the child was born she exposed and laid it down in the head of the Cannongate.' She had spent the next two years in Dundee and then six months in Fife before returning to Aberdeen and being apprehended and imprisoned. An attempt was made to find out what had become of the child but unsuccessfully. As she had so callously abandoned it, 'not takeing care thereof that it might be exposed to great hazard', the Justice Court – which could impose more drastic penalties than the session – appointed her

> to be taken by the hand of the common executioner, and carryed to the fish cross and put in the Jougs there to remain for the space of halfe an hour, And thereafter ordain her to be whipped by the sd Executioner untill she come to the Gallowgate port And banishes her furth and from this burgh & freedome never to return thereto under the pain of being corporally punished.[5]

Kirk sessions had a twofold concern with foundlings. First, there was the moral issue, and second, if the mother could not be traced then the foundling would have to be brought up at the expense of the parish. Old Aberdeen session in August 1705, 'considering that much of the poors money is expended upon the maintenance of the foundlings the session appoynted that nixt Lords day Intimation be made from pulpit that the Congregation extend their Charity upon that account that the poor may not be at so great a loss for the future.' That session made a similar appeal in August 1712, in January 1719, and in February 1726.

The number of foundlings supported by a session at any given time is difficult to get at. South Leith session noted in April 1693 that they had '5 or six upon their hand

4: The Background to Illegitimacy and Bridal Pregnancy

to mentain'.[6] In February 1735 Edinburgh St Cuthbert's session was 'Infested & Burdened with foundlings, Four of whom having been found Exposed in the parish in the space of two moneths.' But the scale of this problem in Edinburgh is revealed in the kirk treasurer's accounts for the year 1741, when no less than 58 foundlings were recorded.[7]

When a foundling was discovered and a nurse had been found for it, the top priority was to try and locate the mother. An announcement would be made from the pulpit in the hope that someone would come forward with information. In November 1719 Old Aberdeen session decided that 'the Drummer should goe through the Town with his Drum for the effect forsaid'. The other ploy which sessions used was to arrange for midwives to see if there was milk in the breasts of any unmarried women in the parish. These ploys rarely succeeded; we estimate that for perhaps 75 per cent of foundlings, the mother was not traced. If she was, it was usually either because the session was already aware of her pregnancy and was keeping an eye on her, or it was because the infant had been left by someone else.

An example of a woman who did not expose her own child is Margaret Ramsay, who appeared before St Cuthbert's session in December 1702. She confessed that her child was begotten in fornication with James Finlay, cordiner, who, along with his sister, 'called for her child in order to give it up to be nursed, and accordingly she gave them the child, but fearing lest they should have slain the child she enquired for him, and found that he was laid down at the westend of the westport'. Another example is Isobell McComrie in South Leith (September 1735). Her child had also been taken from her by its father, 'And when, after her recovery, she found that her child was not in the place where it was said to be sent to, & hearing of a child exposed in Leith, she went to see the same, & knew the child to be her child'. There was an unusual twist to one example of a case where a mother was discovered because the session was already keeping an eye on her. When an exposed child was found in South Leith in October 1734 Janet Pittillo, who had confessed to fornication in May, was suspected to be the mother and was incarcerated in the Tolbooth; she eventually admitted that she had exposed her child but in Edinburgh, so the one in Leith was not hers. Her own child was found in Edinburgh and restored to her.

Sometimes an infant was laid at the door of its putative father. For instance, in Dundee in August 1776 Anne Valentine left her child at the house of John Coutts, her partner in adultery, and disappeared. Coutts' wife then took the infant and left it outside an elder's house. The session decided that 'a Complaint ought to be made to the Provost as Justice of Peace in order that John Coutts may be taken up & oblidged to provide for her child'. Coutts insisted that he was not its father; the belief that a child would be born exactly nine months from the day of fornication led him, in common with others, to deny paternity. In a similar case in North Leith in April 1752 a child was laid down at the door of Isabel Ewan, lately married to David Clerk, sailor, allegedly because its mother had not been given any subsistence by Clerk. Isabel said that Clerk had admitted to her that he had been guilty of fornication with the other woman but had insisted that the child was not his because of the timing of the birth. The session were 'satisfyed that as David Clerk owned guilt with the Mother of this Child... he will in Law be Constructed the father of it; And as the said Isabel Ewan owns her Marriage to the said David... They order her either to keep the Child as she was Married to its Father, or go & seek the Mother, and give the Child to her'. She 'promised to do all in her power to find out the Mother if the Session

57

would assist her, which they promised to do'. In South Leith (November 1722) Mary Dickson left her six-month-old child in the stair of James Robertson, sailor, with the following note:

> James you know that the child is yours, & I have keeped him this half year this same day, & I am sorry to part with him but am not able to keep him any longer for I am in a poor condition at present, God help me, & the childs name is James. I pray you lay it to mind, or I will lay him down to you both before God & Man.

When James returned he promised to take care of the child.

The cost of maintenance was the commonest reason women gave for abandoning a child. In St Cuthbert's (February 1699) Grizel Girdwood confessed laying down her child because 'she was not able to maintain the same, and because one Thomas Colwell in Edinburgh who payed the Child's quarter formerly, refuses now to do it'. The session 'ordered her to make application to the Civil Magistrate for payment thereof, and withall charged her to take back the child'. In the same parish in November 1773 Janet Beaton confessed that she was the mother of a child recently abandoned. She declared that Lord Hume was the father and that she was delivered in October 1772, that a few days before Christmas he gave her five pounds 'with promise of a farther supply But that notwithstanding of several applications she never had received any farther supply from his Lordship'.

Although, inevitably, some foundlings died, if an infant was left at the father's house, or outside the house of an elder, the intention was that it be picked up and cared for. Even in other cases this could be true. Isobel Campbell confessed to St Cuthbert's session in October 1711 that she was the mother of a recently exposed infant. She said that when she left it 'she absconded at a distance till she saw the child taken up by a woman, and then she made her escape'. Grizel Morison, also in St Cuthbert's (January 1721) exposed her child but 'received the child the same day he was Exposed, for her Bowels yearned upon him so that she could not want [do without] him'. However, in a Dundee case (April 1702), a child survived only because of community action. Janet Ramsay stole away with her child

> which when the people perceived they pursued the woman fearing she should murther the chyld & overtook her betwixt Glames & Dundee but she had not the chyld, but when they threatned her she told them the place where she had depositat the chyld so they went altogether to that place and found the chyld alyve and they caused her to tak up the chyld and brought her to Dundie & put her into Bailie Maxwells hand.

As the child was alive there was no need for criminal proceedings, but very occasionally in session registers mention is made of a woman convicted of infanticide. In St Cuthbert's (May 1743) Thomas Forrest was defined as 'the unhappy lad who was the father of the child, for the murther of which Margaret Stewart was lately execute'. Sessions did not normally become involved in such cases as they came under criminal jurisdiction from the outset, but in Old Aberdeen in April 1727 they were forced to do so when Barbara Nicoll claimed to have miscarried but would not produce any evidence. Subsequently she said that the child was born dead and that she buried it. She took some elders to the spot and the body was dug up; some women inspecting it judged that 'the child was come to the mature

4: The Background to Illegitimacy and Bridal Pregnancy

tyme of Birth', so she was handed over to the civil authorities.

A lengthy, and ultimately even more grisly, case came before St Cuthbert's in July 1756. Rabina Gemils claimed to have miscarried after four months of pregnancy. She said that the father was an unknown man who had attacked her, but it was generally believed that her master, William Wallace, was the true father; it was known that Wallace's wife had delivered the child and buried it immediately afterwards. In view of all this the session insisted on being shown where the body was buried. Unfortunately, in raising it 'the body was mangled', but 'they caused part of the body be brought up, and laid in the little Kirk'. Two midwives were asked 'to come and inspect that part of the body which now lyes in the little Kirk, being part of the Skull and the hinderlings of the body'; 'they were of Opinion that the Child seemed to have been at the full time or very near it'. Rabina was committed to prison.

Why, where, and in what circumstances did unmarried women in early modern Scottish cities succumb to men and potential pregnancy? For the 'where', there were some unusual locations. In Leith on more than one occasion it happened on board a ship sailing from London.[8] In August 1776 Janet Douglass confessed to Edinburgh St Cuthbert's session that she had been guilty of fornication with Mr John Newlands, ensign, now in America, saying that it happened only once, after he had called at her father's house and had left a chaise standing at the door

> That she went out with a Candle to light him to the Chaise and that he carried her into the Chaise and drove off with her, that the Guilt was contracted in the Chaise and that Mr Newlands sent her back in the Chaise to her Father's House some little time after he carried her away the same Evening.

But it most often happened in the house where the woman was serving.

The readiest explanation for a fall in fornication is simple proximity. Young men and women were serving together without necessarily any strict supervision over them. In Glasgow Barony (October 1747) Margaret Cochran declared that her child was begotten in her master's house 'in the night time, when the Family were in Bed'. David Anderson, the man she accused, and another male servant shared one bed in the kitchen, while she slept in another, and on the night in question she said that 'the said Anderson left his own Bed, and came to hers and stayed about an hour in Bed with her'. He denied this, but others who had been in the house that night declared that the couple had been in bed together, and 'there was much Noise between them in the way of Shrieking and merryment'.

In October 1786 Robert Hughes appeared before Dundee session on a complaint brought by Robert Martin regarding his son. Hughes 'acknowledged that James Martin his Apprentice & a Servant girl he had did sleep together in one Bed for three Nights & that he thought no harm could arise from it as they were both so young'. Although the ages are not specified, the horror with which the session reacted to this indicates that such naïveté was uncommon. Nevertheless, young servants were frequently in close proximity, with inevitable results.

In the above cases, sex was consensual and, one assumes, enjoyable. But in November 1711 Margaret Farquhar complained to North Leith session of Thomas Hay, son of her mistress. She had been obliged 'to leave her service' because of his constant harassment, and since then 'the said Thomas continues his importunity threatning to do her harm when he can have a fitt occasion, but that she had hitherto escap'd his malicious design, and humbly desired that the said Thomas might be restrain'd from the like for the future'. Thomas 'judicially confessed that he had offered to committ uncleanness with the said Margaret, which he did in sport, but had no design of harm to her'. (Margaret also complained that Thomas's mother had 'rated' her for going to the minister about this; the latter confessed that 'in her passion she had emitted some rash expressions'.)

Margaret was unusual in evading the attentions of the man in question. Much more typical was the case of Elizabeth Porteous, who appeared before Edinburgh St Cuthbert's session after having an illegitimate child in July 1744, saying that the father was her master's son and that 'she was forced by said John against her will when there was no body in the house'. Or Margaret Miller, who told South Leith session (November 1708) that Robert Allan, skipper, stayed in her master's house on the night of 2 May and asked her to carry a candle to his room; when they got there 'he threw her over on the bed & took both her Armes & put them on her mouth so that she could not get spoken'. She added that 'on the Morrow she reproved him for what he had done to her and that he put his hands behind his back & laughed in her face'. In a particularly nasty incident Elizabeth Falconer (South Leith, October 1733) said that John Greenfield, shipmaster, 'dragged her down her Masters stair, & not only had carnal dealling with her himself, but also held her & stopped her mouth, till George Paris also had carnal dealling with her.' Both men later confessed; the word 'rape' was not mentioned.

Examples could be multiplied. In Old Aberdeen (July 1698) Margaret Fiddes accused William Murray, '& did instance what measures he took to prevaill with her to gratifie his carnall & sinfull desyres, in sending for her while she was in Bed severall tymes'. She had always refused, but once in the daytime, 'not thinking upon any evil', she 'came to him, and how soon she entered his Chamber, he assaulted her so vigorously, that there was no possibility of escapeing, though she endeavoured to the utmost of her power & cryed for assistance but to no purpose, they being in ane outhouse... besydes she declared that in his struglaing with her he abused her so inhumanely That for a considerable tyme thereafter she did spitt blood, & kept bed immediately thereafter.' In Edinburgh St Cuthbert's (May 1707) Elspeth Milne named John Mcintosh, a married man, and said that 'she cry'd for help'. He denied guilt, but a witness declared that 'she saw John Mcintosh pull Elspeth Milne by the arm into his house, and when they were in the house, the door was closs shutt upon them, and when Elspeth came out of the house, the Deponent heard her say Devill take him away filthy fellow, and her countenance was dejected, and she seemed to be weeping.'

In rural parishes the head of the household in which a woman served was likely to be of the same social class as herself. In towns there was likely to be a much greater disparity, and therefore a much higher level of intimidation. In the majority of cases where a woman declared that she had been forced into intercourse the man was her master, and married. Margaret Boiswal told St Cuthbert's session (March 1733) that the father of her child was William Campbell: 'when they were guilty there was none present in the family save themselves, her mistress & the nurse with the Child being absent, and about four of the afternoon he coming upon her in a surprize, and taking her by the waist she resisting him did at first shake herself free of him, but no person being near he at length overcame her, and threw her into the Green bed of the

4: The Background to Illegitimacy and Bridal Pregnancy

Kitchen where the nurse lyes, and committed Lewdness with her'.

What is shocking to the modern reader is the realisation that in all of the above cases the unwilling woman was considered as guilty as the man. (And as the penalty was the same whether she was willing or not, there was no reason for her to lie.) This was partly because a woman's claim of having been 'forced' was uncorroborated, but mainly because it was believed that, whatever the circumstances, it was a woman's responsibility to make certain that such a thing did not happen. Only one woman dared to question this, and it did not do her any good. In December 1744 St Cuthbert's session ordered Marion Mitchell, a widow, to appear publicly for her sin with James Borthwick, 'whereupon she signified that she could not think of appearing publickly in regard she was compelled by him to this sin being alone in her house'. The ministers were to 'endeavour to bring her to some sense of her Iniquity', but it was reported at the January meeting that she had not been to see them. 'The session inclining to show her all the favour they can, on account of a Representation made of her former good character' referred it to the elders in her bounds to deal with her. In February she was referred to the presbytery as contumacious, but by the end of March she bowed to pressure and submitted to discipline for her 'guilt'.

In view of this treatment of an innocent victim, it is not so surprising that Jane Menzies, a member of the gentry class (daughter of the deceased Menzies of Kenmudie) fled from discipline at Aberdeen after bearing her bastard child in January 1747. The father was 'one Polwarth a Serjeant in the Regiment call'd the Old Buffs... in her father's house in this town the day before the Duke of Cumberland with the Army went north', when 'the said Polwarth forced and ravished her, stopping her mouth with his Napkin'.[9]

We found only one case where an accusation of rape resulted in a woman being cleared (though the man was still not called a rapist). In Aberdeen (January 1744) Elizabeth Dason complained that George Smith, her master, had ravished her; he denied the charge. The circumstance that made all the difference was that a few days before it happened Elizabeth told neighbours that her master 'had been attempting to lye carnally with her' and asked their advice. One 'answer'd that she should tell the Story before him and his wife and then his wife would cause him forbear such Attempts in time coming.' Another had 'advis'd her to resist his Attempts and if he offer'd again, to tell her Mistress and leave their Service.' Because the testimony of those witnesses proved that she had done her best to evade his attentions the presbytery dismissed Elizabeth from discipline and ordered Smith to satisfy as an adulterer.

The economic situation of a woman servant made it difficult to stop working for a man, no matter how he behaved. Margaret Walls told Dundee session in December 1762 that her master, John Brown of Glanvell, 'came into the Kitchen on the Fifth Day of July last in the afternoon, and after using Intreaties in vain, he cut the Cloaths off her, and lay with her by Force, that there was no person but themselves in the house, and that he dragged her into his own Room before he lay with her... As soon as she could get free of him which was a little before Eight o clock at night, she immediately left his house and went to Elizabeth Duncan, the woman who had feed her to Mr Brown, and told said Elizabeth Duncan what had happened and the usage she had got.' Elizabeth later told the session that Margaret had showed her 'a Black petticoat, cut on the Top of the right side by Mr Brown with his penknife'. Elizabeth

Sin in the City

had gone to see Brown and asked him why Margaret had left his service: 'He answered she had no reason but went away in a Freak', and told Elizabeth to bring her back, but Margaret 'positively refused to return'. Margaret clearly had a strong case, but in May when she was called before the session she did not appear, which suggests that she had succumbed to pressure by Brown. The session, considering that she 'had brought in a heavy Charge against John Brown of Glanvell, but that the Evidence she adduced was by no means a proof of its Truth, and that she compeared not when legally summoned, to hear Sentence, They found her liable to Censure.'

Apart from proximity and intimidation there was another reason why a woman might succumb to a man, and that was the hope of marriage. 'Failed courtship' is the term used for women who get pregnant in the hope or expectation of marriage, but a promise of marriage was not often claimed in our cities. In Edinburgh Trinity College in the 1670s over a fifth of the women put forward this justification; by the 1690s it had disappeared. In St Cuthbert's it was about 17 per cent in the 1660s and in most decades later there were a few instances, all together about 5 per cent of the cases. In South Leith there was a steady small number, between 3 and 5 per cent of all cases. In both the Aberdeen parishes the instances were negligible. Glasgow Barony had no cases at all, and Govan very few, except in the 1760s when for some inexplicable reason some 12 per cent of women claimed a promise of marriage. On the whole, it seems that promises of marriage were seldom part of the process of seduction.

In any case, such a hope was often forlorn. In South Leith (August 1694) George McCaulla, the father of Katherine Nisbet's dead child, had also fathered her previous child (dead too) as well as another woman's bastard. Katherine said that both her children had been begotten under promise of marriage, '& the promise severall tymes renewed'.

One might have thought that a woman committing adultery would not do so with any hope of marriage, but Isobel Lillie (South Leith December 1731) said that John McCay 'gave her many inticeing words, particularly, that he told her that his wife was a dying woman, & that he would marry her upon the death of his wife'. McCay's wife subsequently did die, but far from marrying Isobel he denied to the session 'that ever he gave her a kiss of his mouth'. The session did not believe him, and there was some poetic justice in this case, for she left the child behind her as a foundling, and the session decided that 'seeing he had let the mother slip, he behoved to ease the session of the burden of maintaining the child'. A familiar lament was made by Grizel Morison in St Cuthbert's (October 1720). She was the servant of a widower and declared that 'it was upon promise of marriage that she yeelded to him, he at that time Imprecating that he might be like Lot's Wife turn'd into a pillar of salt if he did not marry her, and this was before they sinned and after commiting of the Lewdness he never cared for her'.

Sympathy was shown by Aberdeen session toward Katherine Fillan (Nov 1782) who declared that John Mcpherson, the father of her child, 'enticed her under pretence of Courtship and promise of marriage and had gone so far as to fix the latter end of June for their intended marriage, That he declared to her he had been a farmer in the north Country, and that he was then going to settle on part of a farm betwixt Peterhead & Fraserburgh'. He had also told her 'that he was a Widower, and that his wife had dyed sometime ago in the old Town'. Although Mcpherson was never tracked down, her story was believed, and when she applied to be allowed to satisfy

4: The Background to Illegitimacy and Bridal Pregnancy

discipline in 1784 ('as she was deeply sensible of her sin & folly and grievously affected with the hard lot she was under by being cut off from Church privileges or sealing ordinances on that Account'), she was not made to satisfy for adultery but was in fact let off with a sessional rebuke.

One of the saddest stories was that of Janet Clark, late servant and housekeeper to George Cramond, brewer, in Dundee, who had been forced to take drugs to abort her child, as related above. Cramond 'came to her Bedside in the Kitchen, when she was sleeping alone – that upon her crying out he started and retired a little, but afterwards returned and carried her to the Bed, & was then & there guilty of uncleanness with her.' A fortnight later, she said, it happened again; 'what led her into a Compliance the Second Time was his promising to marry her, which promise he continued afterward to repeat.' About a month later she fainted, and Cramond said he would get something from the doctor, '& that if she would take the Drugs he should get for her, then he would afterwards marry her.' After appearing before the session and telling them the story Janet wrote to Cramond, saying that 'if he would fulfill his promise to her she would be a good Wife to him, and that this would all die down.' His response was to advise her 'to deny all she had confessed to the session & he would make it up with her afterwards.' This she refused to do. In January a witness told the session that he had recently told Janet 'that her Master was going to be married; That thereupon she burst into Tears... That as she was then threatening to destroy herself, they earnestly entreated her to lay aside such unchristian Thoughts.'

Another Dundee abortion case related earlier in this chapter was also a deluded hope of marriage. Marjory Thoms had already borne one child to James Ross, and she had told him afterwards

> that she thought that he ought to keep at a distance from her – to which he answered that he never would keep at a distance from her while he was alive & accordingly deluded her in such a manner upon the terms of Marriage – that he came once or twice a Week to her Room till she was seven Months gone with her last Child to him – that she then insisted with him to let her know what he meant to do in regard to his marrying her as her being with Child could be no longer concealed – that he then said he would come back next friday & consult that matter & would come & drink Tea.

It was on that occasion that he slipped various substances into her food and drink in the attempt to have her abort.

However, there were some genuine promises of marriage. When Katherine Thomson appeared before Edinburgh New Kirk session in March 1711 she named William Innes, barber, as father of her unborn child. He was now in London, but she produced a letter signed by both of them: 'This I give you under my hand to you Katherine Thomson That I shall never have another woman in this world But you wherever I am there you will come to me, This you promise to Me also to be my Loveing wife, And I also to be your Loveing husband God willing'. As he had left the parish before she realised she was pregnant the session still demanded an acknowledgement of paternity and in June she produced another letter from him admitting guilt and mentioning 'his resolutions for marieing her when he returns'.

Even when there was a disparity in social classes the possibility of marriage still existed. Aberdeen session did not believe Isobel Moir in March 1722 when she named Mr Andrew Livingstone, late Episcopal minister, as father of her unborn child. They warned her 'to be ware of wronging any man, particularly a man that had the character of a Minister'. She alleged a promise of marriage, made 'in a solemn way', and said that she had left his service with a view to arranging their marriage. By the beginning of May, when he appeared to acknowledge the truth of her allegation, the sin was antenuptial fornication, for they were married.

Antenuptial fornication – or bridal pregnancy, as we would call it – was considered a lesser sin than fornication not followed by marriage, but a sin none the less. Most sessions required only one public appearance by the couple, though Dundee required three. It was easy enough to establish, since at the time of first birth the marriage register could be consulted. In the seventeenth century some sessions required couples to pay a consignation fee which would be returned if a child was not born within nine months.

The aim of sessions to persuade those guilty of antenuptial fornication to make their public appearance could lead to more difficulties than for ordinary fornication. Having achieved 'respectability' a woman, in particular, was anything but keen to be publicly humiliated in front of the congregation for a fall before marriage. If the birth took place some seven months after the wedding she might claim that it was premature.

For example, two couples appeared before St Cuthbert's session in September 1700, both denying antenuptial fornication. Helen Kerr said that she 'gott a stress by washing which hastened the birth of her child'. Elders spoke with the midwife and women present at the birth who declared that 'the child was compleat in all its parts'; both couples confessed shortly after that. In October 1738 Marian Anderson declared to North Leith session that 'she was delivered before her due time by some hurt she had received'. The midwife was called, and the couple, 'failing in proof of their Exculpation Judicially Confessed their Guilt'. A Dundee midwife refused to assist the session with their enquiry into a premature delivery in April 1702. 'That was non of her business', she responded, 'goe ask the parent'. However, expert witnesses could be useful in providing evidence that a child was not full term. In October 1704 one such witness declared to St Cuthbert's session that Jane Burd's newborn infant had been 'very weak & small, and wanted nails both upon her fingers & toes'. The session decided 'to proceed no further in the affair'.

A different category was a child born after a woman was married, which her husband disowned. We did not count such births in our illegitimacy figures, as legally the child was not a bastard, but naturally sessions treated women in these cases as ordinary fornicators. Old Aberdeen session (July 1682) dealt with Isobel Grant, married to James Jameson but bearing a child to Alexander Leith, 'the said Isobel knowing her selfe to be with chyld to the said Alexander at the tyme she was married with the said James Jameson who was altogether Ignorant of the thing'.

In December 1738 when Elizabeth Bishop had her first child, she told St Cuthbert's session that she was guilty with her husband, Archbald Shaw, in May, before their marriage, and he confessed the same. Being asked if she had been guilty with any other man, she replied that in March 'a young Gentleman... attack'd and abus'd her'. She was then asked 'how she came to marry the man now her husband, and had another man's child in her belly, Answer'd that she never suspected the child was any other body's than the man now her Husband, till the [date of the] Birth discover'd it.' Naming an 'unknown gentleman' as father of one's child normally meant appearing as an adulteress, but in this case 'the session from their tender

4: The Background to Illegitimacy and Bridal Pregnancy

regard to her now in her married state, require of her only to appear three several Lord's days'; her husband was to share the final appearance with her. St Cuthbert's session in May 1776 felt much less sympathy for Alison Short who gave birth to one man's child nine weeks after being married to another. She was not allowed absolution at that time because of 'the aggravating circumstances of her guilt and the injury done to her Husband'.

As mentioned above, we counted such cases as bridal pregnancies; there must have been other children accepted by a husband who were not in truth of his begetting. This came to light in the case of Isobel Henderson (Dundee, June 1762) only because 'while in Distress and likely to die, [she] declared to her Husband and some others, that Child of which she was delivered in Summer last, was not her husband's, as was then supposed, but that the Child was begotten by another Man sometime before she was married to David Craig'. She then recovered and appeared before the session, confessing that when she married Craig, she was two months gone with child to George Patullo

> and that in six months and about two or three Days after her Marriage, she had brought forth the Child, which she pretended was born in the seventh month, and at that Time asserted that it was her husband's in order to conceal her shame: But that being lately in Distress, and at the point of Death, her Conscience, burdened with a sense of Guilt, obliged her to confess it to her Husband, and others, before God, in order that she might obtain Mercy.

Of course, many cases of antenuptial fornication were perfectly straightforward, just as were many cases of illegitimacy. However, the wealth of detail recorded in kirk session records has meant that we have been able to gain valuable insight into the circumstances in which children were begotten outwith marriage.

Notes

Edinburgh, Canongate and Leith kirk session registers are in the Scottish Record Office; the only exception is Edinburgh New Kirk which for the year 1706 is in Edinburgh University Library and for several other years in Edinburgh City Archive. Aberdeen St Nicholas registers are in Aberdeen City Archive; Old Machar registers are in the parish church, with access via Aberdeen University – microfilms of both sessions' records are in the Scottish Record Office. Glasgow Barony and Govan session registers are in Glasgow City Archive, and have not been microfilmed. Dundee registers are in Dundee City Archive, with microfilms in Edinburgh. We have not given references for each citation but always state the month and year, making it possible for anyone to find a particular case.

1 The first mention of the bond which we found was in Trinity College October 1702. Alison Alexander had assisted Grissell Kyll, whose child was begotten in Liberton parish. The midwife was asked why she had not informed the minister or elder of the bounds and said that the woman in whose house this took place had done so. 'Being asked if she hath subt the Bond with the rest of the Midwives, she answered no'.
2 North Leith was rather different. Here, between 1711 and 1720, 21 per cent of women were discovered after five months and 21 per cent after their child was born, while in the 1730s 41 per cent were cited under five months pregnant, while only one woman had already borne her child. However, with samples of only 19 and 17 the numbers are too far small to

Sin in the City

allow serious comparisons.
3. In May 1779 Aberdeen had another such case. Christian Hutcheon had left the parish and was reported to have been pregnant at the time which she denied. The session received a letter from an elder in Peterhead, declaring that 'she had been bad in her health while at her Mothers house'. The session found 'there were no presumptions of Guilt' against her and therefore considered the report 'as groundless and dismiss the process, and appoint an Extract hereof to be given her by the Clerk for her vindication.'
4. Gray fled soon afterwards, and no evidence of her having venereal disease was produced. However, in the same session in September 1730 Agnes Johnston delated herself guilty of adultery with James Dove, not because she was pregnant but because 'she thought she had gott the Clap from him for she could neither goe nor work, and she never knew any man carnally save James Dove, who when he saw her crippleing Up and Down the year he bad her to take warm water to bath herself & the blades of Beets to apply to her Sores to give her ease.' And in Dundee in June 1792 Catherine Macleod said that the father of her child 'infected her with the Venereal Disease', which was confirmed by the midwife.
5. Aberdeen Justice Court records are in Aberdeen City Archive.
6. The session was going to ask the Lord Advocate 'whither or not the hous rents or other fortunes of a deserter may be applyed for the mentainance of his deserted Child'. In April 1694 the session petitioned the Privy Council for money to maintain 'severall fondlings laid doun which belong to soldiers that goe to flanders'.
7. Edinburgh Kirk Treasurer's accounts are in Edinburgh City Archive. The list is of 'Cash payed for Nursing & keeping Foundlings & Orphans'. Orphans are named while foundlings are just listed as 'a Foundling' with the name of the person to whom payment was made. When a name is repeated we have assumed that additional payment was being made for the same foundling and counted it only once.
8. In June 1694 Charles Vans, seaman, confessed that Grizzell Waterstoun's accusation of him as father was true. The session thought he should satisfy church discipline in their church as she had done 'becaus they found the sin was committed in a ship belonging to Leith and that the scandall broke furth in this place'. Vans 'absolutely refused' and was referred to the presbytery.
9. She was not the only Aberdeen victim of the Forty Five. Margaret Walker was married to Peter Hervie in June 1746, but when her child was born in December he would not own it as his. She declared that in March 'she was forced & ravished by one Samson Pierce or Piece a Serjeant in the Regiment called the Old Buffs, in her own dwelling house'. Amazingly, the following March she was able to produce a letter 'from Samson Pearce acknowledging himself to be the father of her Child'.

Appendix 1

Bond signed by midwives
Edinburgh St Cuthbert's parish, 12 December 1718

Be it known to all men by these presents We Helen Bulloch spouse to Edward Hill freeman Cordiner in Portsburgh Mary Ferguson spouse to Mark Harries Tanner there, Agnes Robertson Spouse to John Wallace Cordiner there, Janet McGrigor Spouse to Thomas Paterson Cordiner in Potter-row, Jane Wallace spouse to William Anderson Weaver in the Water of Leith, Sarah Martin Spouse to James Sharp Indweller in Dalry-milns, Helen Oar Relict of Dorret Indweller in Ninians row Rachel Turnbull Indweller in Canon-milns midwives in the parish of Westkirk Forasmuch as there are several women in the said parish who of late have brought forth Children in Uncleanness, and tho' much pains have been taken upon them, to bring them to confess who are the fathers of their Children, yet they obstinatly refuse to give an account of them, they still alledging that they were gott with child in open fields by persons they never saw before, and there are others also who give up false fathers to their Children and other strumpets also who are guilty of Exposing their children brought forth in uncleanness. Therefore... we by the Tenor herof Bind and Oblige us the said Midwives of the Westkirk parish to perform these Rules following First That at all times we shall serve the poor in our occupation when required. Secondly that we shall at no time whatsomever administer drugs to any woman with child without advice of a physician, Thirdly That we shall give an Account of all unlawfull Births which come to our knowledge within the said parish to the Ministers or Elders of the Bounds where these births happen and that within the space of Four hours before or after, and if it shall happen that if the mother vary anent the child's father or we have any suspicious therof, that we shall call for the said ministers or Elders in time of Labour, or in their absences for two habile Witnesses in the Neighbourhood, and thoroughly examine the Mother before child bearing in order to oblige her to give an impartiall account of the Child's Father, and we shall neither conceal, nor concurr in concealing of the father or mother of any child so brought forth in the said parish Fourthly that we shall very willingly meet with other midwives at the Magistrates of Justices of peace their order anent Foundlings or undiscovered Births of any such like occurring in the said parish, and shall give personall attendance therupon in the way of our Imployment Fifthly that we shall discover to the magistrates or Justices aforsaid all persons within the said parish who at present or hereafter to our knowledge shall take upon them the office of a midwife who have not subscribed these presents, and are not approven by the Magistrates and Justices of peace as they shall appoint & Sixthly that we shall faithfully discharge our duty in our offices respective and use our utmost diligence for the safe delivery

Sin in the City

preservation & well-fare of every mother and child which shall come under our care And so oft as we shall fail in the performance of any of the saids Rules we bind & oblige each of us for our selves to pay to Baillie James Adamson or Baillie Andrew Thomson present magistrates of West or East Portsburgh or their successors in office The summ of Twenty pounds scots money for the use of the poor of the said Westkirk paroch.

5

Illegitimacy and Bridal Pregnancy

In January 1693 Old Aberdeen session found that 'the Register of baptisms & burialls belonging to this Church is deficient and many blanks in it'. This was because 'none or very few of the people did ever come to the Clerk to have their Children or friends names registered but always went to the bedall who collected the dues both for the Clerk & himself & it might be supposed that the officer or bedall forsaid might conceal from the Clerk some of those burials or baptisms for his own advantage'. In Edinburgh's West Kirk (St Cuthbert's) parish in November 1743 there were many complaints about the outgoing session clerk (who was deposed for embezzling some of the poor's money). It was discovered that 'in about a third part of the Paroch and in the space of about four years, there is Missing in the Register fifty four Baptisms for any of which Mr Wilson does not so much as pretend to account for':

> As for the Misnaming of Parents & their Children and of the Residence of the Parents, and also the sexes of Children, Males being put for Females, & contra, they find that as Mr Wilson makes no defence for it, so it's highly injurious to the particular persons concerned and hurtfull to the Registers in General.

It may be inferred from the above extracts that the usefulness of Old Parish Registers for this (or any other) purpose in our period is very limited. Old Parish Registers have been used for the measurement of illegitimacy in England. There is a study covering a large number of parishes from 1538–1754.[1] The figures derived depend on the reliability of parish clerks in noting the absence of married parents at the registration of baptism, and there is a risk of under registration and of failure to note. These risks means that illegitimacy is likely to be understated.

Session registers are clearly preferable, since discipline, which occupied a large part of the time of the sessions, was seen as an essential activity for a Christian community. We have done our best to calculate the illegitimacy ratio, that is the percentage of births that were by unmarried women. We have also tried to find the percentage of women who had more than one illegitimate child ('repeaters'), those who were pregnant when they were married, and those for whom their first conception was outwith wedlock. But there are difficulties in using the discipline record to get estimates the levels of sexual misbehaviour in the different towns. For one thing, as can be seen from Appendix 2, only a limited number of kirk session registers appear to have survived for Edinburgh parishes, and none at all for central Glasgow until after our period.

Another difficulty in to establish the denominator, i.e. the total births for any particular decade. Since we cannot rely on the Old Parish Registers, we have attempted to get probable levels of births from the scale of the urban population. We have some idea of the population of our towns in the 1690s from the records of the hearth and poll taxes. Particularly detailed studies have been made of Aberdeen and Edinburgh in the late seventeenth century. We have Webster's figures for 1755, and Webster has increasingly commanded the respect of historical demographers. We have the figures in the *Statistical Account* for the early 1790s. Occasionally there are other figures which are convincing, such as those in the South Leith ministers' catechising records for the middle decades of the eighteenth century.[2]

These figures can be used to give probable levels for births. The recent analysis of Webster's age distribution produced a birth rate of just over 36 per thousand annual births.[3] We calculated birth levels on the assumption that the Webster figure obtained in the cities throughout our period. This probably gives too high a level of births, bearing in mind the relatively high proportion of young adults in servant status and not free to marry, and as a result understates the illegitimacy percentage. If the birth rate stood at 30 per thousand, the level of illegitimacy would be approximately a fifth higher than is shown in our figures.

As in our earlier study,[4] we collected the figures for unmarried women 'delated' (reported) to the session as being 'with child' or having been delivered of a child. The reporting of such women was done by the elders of each city district. The woman would be cited to appear before the session where she would be asked the name of the man responsible.

We collected those cases by decades. If the record of a year does not appear complete we have omitted that year, and we have not recorded a decade which did not appear to have five complete years. In the case of the fragmented material from several of the central parishes in Edinburgh (Old Kirk, New Kirk, Old and New Greyfriars, and Lady Yester's), we have collected the scraps which can be found but have not used them as a quantifiable source. For Aberdeen our figures come from the session register but, as shown in Chapter 2, the justice court of Aberdeen carried some cases which did not come before the session, and the session also has cases which were missed by the justice court. Therefore our figures for Aberdeen, and almost certainly for the Edinburgh parishes of Canongate and Trinity College cannot be regarded as complete.

We attempted to stick to the rules that we had made for our rural study in order to provide a direct comparison. The first was that we ascribed illegitimate births to the parish where the couples made their penitential appearances in the parish church, regardless of where the child was born. Kirk sessions normally confined their disciplinary activity to cases in which conception was believed to have taken place in the parish unless considerable scandal had arisen in the new parish of residence. As will be clear from the previous chapter, in city parishes this meant a number of cases being referred to other sessions, either neighbouring city ones or rural ones. We certainly found a higher level of sessions attempting to transfer responsibility for pregnant unmarried women in city parishes than we did in rural parishes. An obvious point to be made in this respect is that the actual number of illegitimate births in any of our towns would be considerably higher if they were taken from any kind of register of births than from kirk session discipline cases. Our methodology therefore illuminates the success or otherwise of social control in our cities rather than the number of illegitimate children born within them.

As in our earlier study, we recorded twins only when the register explicitly referred to a double birth, and we therefore probably missed some multiple births. We made no allowance for stillbirths and counted all births where the mother

5: Illegitimacy and Bridal Pregnancy

claimed the child had been born dead. However, when it was reported that a mother had miscarried ('parted with child' was the phrase used) we did not count the birth.

We did not count any case where the mother was a married woman, even when the father was definitely not her husband, since the child would not be legally defined as a bastard.[5] In retrospect it might have been useful to have noted these women in a separate category, as they were very much more prevalent in city parishes than in rural ones. Sessions had particular problems with women who claimed that their absent husbands were dead, as the sessions did not know whether to treat the women as fornicators or adulterers and sometimes waited years for proof of a husband's death before proceeding. We followed the session's decisions and included women labelled fornicators while excluding those labelled adulterers. We obviously missed numbering some where a judgment was not made in the surviving record. Women giving birth to a child but claiming an irregular marriage with an absent man proved to be another problem to urban kirk sessions – and to anyone attempting to quantify illegitimate births. Again, if the session believed in the marriage then so did we. Those cases not resolved within the decade obviously had to be excluded by us, which again will have meant under counting.

We have assumed that the discipline record correctly noted when a woman had a second, third or fourth illegitimate child, in modern language 'repeaters'. We collected also the number of male repeaters. We also noted the number of cases where a married couple admitted bridal pregnancy. To obtain a rough figure for the percentage of women whose first conception took place outwith wedlock we combined the number of illegitimate births with the figure for bridal pregnancy and then deducted the number of repeater cases. We assumed that the proportion of births that were firsts in a marriage to be the same as those found in the remarkably full old parish register of Kilmarnock from 1740–1790, one in four, and set our figures of unmarried conception against a quarter of estimated annual births.[6] We are surely safe in concluding that no couple would go through penance for 'antenuptial uncleanness' unless they had truly had sexual intercourse before marriage. Even so there would be couples whose first child managed to postpone birth till after nine months from marriage even if conceived before marriage, so our figures of first conceptions out of wedlock are bound to be too low.

The figures obtained for the percentage of first conceptions taking place out of wedlock contain too many assumptions for much weight to be placed on them. But the high level in some urban parishes is interesting, since almost certainly antenuptial conceptions were under counted. South Leith's figure in the 1760s and 1680s was over 35 per cent and Old Aberdeen's in the late seventeenth century over 40 per cent. By contrast, rural Govan never reached 20 per cent. The striking feature is the contrast in trends between thoroughly urban parishes such as Trinity College, and parishes such as Barony and St Cuthbert's which became urbanised in the later decades of our study. The falling figures in the urbanised parishes almost certainly indicate failure on the part of the session to investigate all cases rather than a genuine change in sexual practices. In Trinity College the instances fell from 56 per cent in the 1660s to 19 per cent in the 1710s, in St Cuthbert's, which seems to have become urbanised early, from 22 per cent in the 1660s to 6 per cent in the 1720s; in Barony (where discipline was maintained until the end of our period) it *rose* from 11 per cent in the 1680s to 19 per cent in the 1760s.

This sample shows that when we have obtained a sequence of figures, decade by decade, it would be rash to assume that they necessarily tell the true story. As the cities expanded and as the business of harbours grew, it became hard for a session to know all that was going on. The rise of irregular marriage created an expanding area of doubt for it hampered the efforts of the sessions to trace the details of cases. Religious dissent existed from the change to presbyterianism of 1690, and became a bigger matter with the rise of presbyterian sects in the second half of the eighteenth century. A fall in discipline cases may reflect the weakening of the discipline system, a drop in the level of extra-marital sex or the establishment of a dissenting congregation. In the later eighteenth century the urbanisation of what had been the rural parishes of Edinburgh St Cuthbert's and Glasgow Barony made it impossible for those sessions to keep up with what was going on. Our estimated illegitimacy ratios and first conceptions out of wedlock decline sharply in almost all our parishes at some point in the eighteenth century, and we conclude that it is at this time that the record parts company with reality.

In the same way the sharp fall in recorded levels of illegitimacy shown in various parishes at different dates, the 1690s (Trinity College), the 1700s (Aberdeen) and the 1710s (South Leith and Old Aberdeen) are unlikely to represent a genuine change in sexual behaviour (see Figures 5.1 and 5.2).

The town that produces the most convincing figures and which does not display a sudden drop is Dundee. The tone of the city's register gives confidence that discipline was kept up into and beyond the 1780s, and that if it was incomplete in say the 1770s, then it had also been so in earlier decades. As can be seen from Figure 5.3, on either estimate of the birth rate, illegitimacy in Dundee was almost always below 4 per cent of births, and in the 1740s and 1750s it sank to just a little over 2 per cent. The pattern in Dundee is very similar to that we found for the neighbouring area of Fife in our earlier study. Also, as in Fife, Dundee had a consistently relatively high level of bridal pregnancy, so that the level there of first conceptions out of wedlock ranged from 8 per cent up to 20 per cent. The general trend of both figures was gently downwards until the 1760s when it was replaced by a gentle rise.

Dundee kept up discipline to the end of the eighteenth century and beyond, but with some difficulties and failures which means that the record is not complete. An important source of weakness is shown in a case of irregular baptism in May 1782, when the father admitted that he had attended dissenting services 'on Account of his not being able to pay for a seat in the established Church'. Pew rents in the cities were decided by the town council, not by the Church, and they have been shown to have deterred working-class attendance in the early nineteenth century,[7] but this instance shows that they were already an obstacle to participation earlier.

We cannot estimate the cases of illegitimacy and bridal pregnancy in the late decades of the eighteenth century, but the gentle rise shown in our figures is surely an understatement. In particular the rise in irregular marriage in Dundee (107 cases in the 1770s in contrast to 31 in the 1760s) makes it unlikely that all bridal pregnancies were noted in the years after 1780. In the 1780s the position of the session resembles that of a voluntary society: only sinners who behaved with proper penitence were allowed to go through the process by which they were reconciled to the Church. In December 1781 a special effort was made to persuade a long list of male adulterers to 'make public satisfaction'. Most refused, and as a result 21 were laid under the sentence of lesser excommunication. But the rise of dissent had robbed this sentence of its terror.

5: Illegitimacy and Bridal Pregnancy

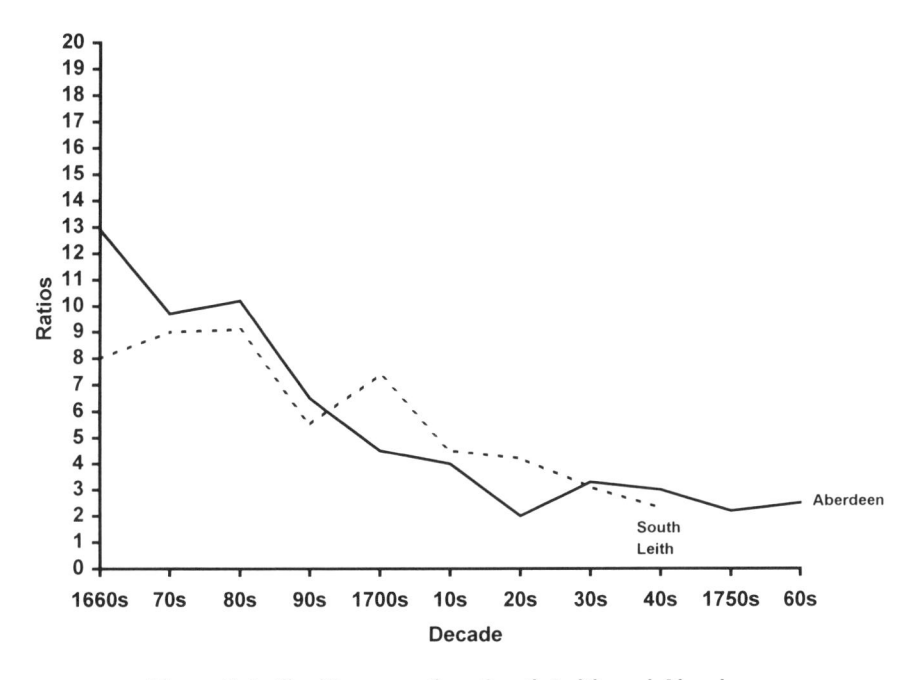

Figure 5.1: Illegitimacy ratios: South Leith and Aberdeen

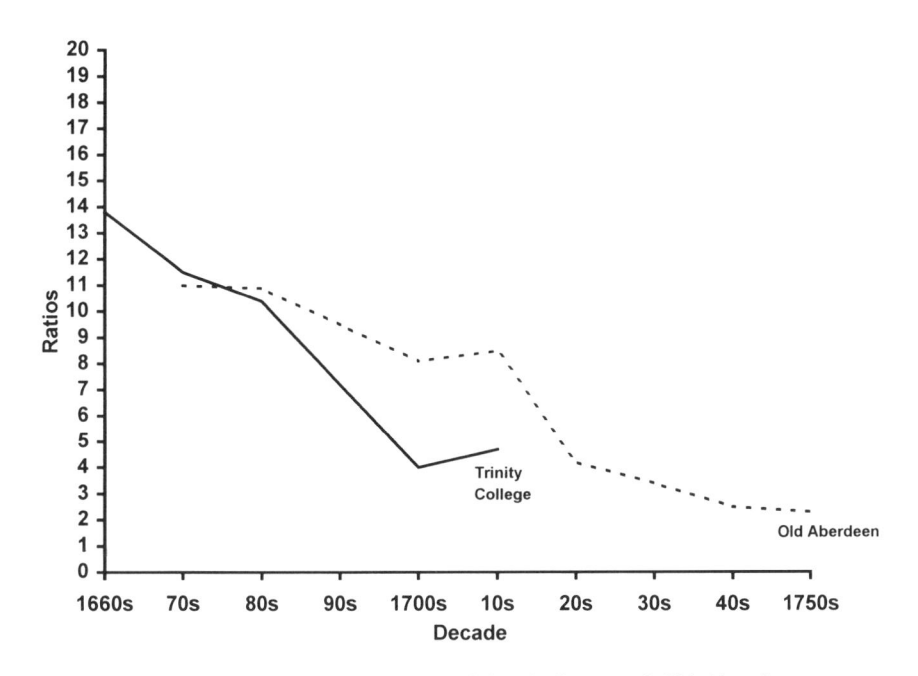

Figure 5.2: Illegitimacy ratios: Trinity College and Old Aberdeen

73

Sin in the City

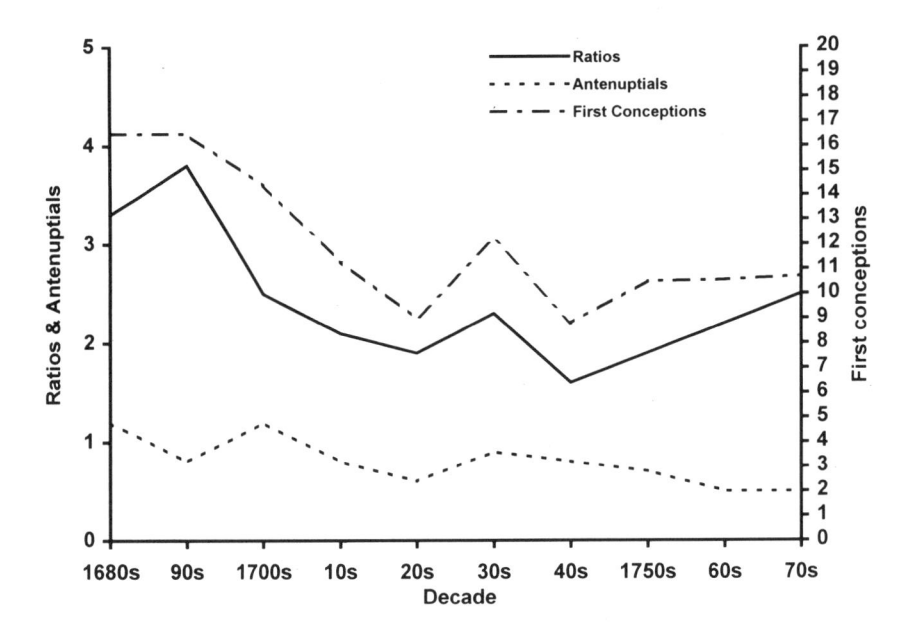

Figure 5.3: Illegitimacy ratios: Dundee

That Dundee still retained the acceptance of discipline into mid-century is shown by the relatively high proportion of men who admitted fornication. Though this was never as high as in the seventeenth century, as late as the 1770s the figure was only just short of half. In this feature Dundee differs from South Leith, which rarely achieved half its men admitting and never rose to the general average of 60 per cent, and from Aberdeen where the level of admissions slumped permanently in the 1740s (see Table 5.1).

Table 5.1: Admission percentages

	Aberdeen	Dundee	South Leith
1660s	70.3	-	46.2
1670s	66.0	-	46.6
1680s	59.0	89.2	54.4
1690s	26.7	94.5	50.6
1700s	89.4	74.0	45.2
1710s	65.0	53.3	38.5
1720s	75.9	66.1	54.4
1730s	51.5	64.3	58.1
1740s	30.8	67.0	37.0
1750s	28.6	59.6	36.4
1760s	40.6	49.1	39.3
1770s	19.6	49.0	25.0

5: Illegitimacy and Bridal Pregnancy

The thorough and careful work of DesBrisay on Aberdeen gives us figures which, even if not absolutely complete, command respect both for the total baptisms and for the cases of fornication in the late seventeenth century. It is these that we have used for the period 1661–1690 in Figure 5.1. His cases are those that came before the justice court, and these exceed those that came before the session by 18 per cent. This is a useful warning that even a source which appears to be thorough and careful may be incomplete. But as noted above, there are cases in the kirk session registers which do not appear in that of the justice court. Both sources may miss the fact that one or other of the sinners is a repeater. For instance in March 1685 Margaret Rolland and John Mackie appear in the justice court as first time sinners, but the session in the same month noted her as a repeater. In October 1685 the justice court dealt with Marjorie Kilgower and George Hedderwick noting her as a repeater. The case got to the session in November but no note was made of the repeat. (It was rare for a session to miss a woman repeater.) The justice court material shows that the session material must always be seen as an understatement of offences of all kinds.

On DesBrisay's figures illegitimacy in Aberdeen between 1661 and 1687 varied between 9.7 per cent and 14 per cent of total births. This is far higher than in rural Aberdeenshire, which ranged between 6 per cent and 8.4 per cent, or the north east rural area where it ranged between 7 per cent and 9.7 per cent. Still, the relatively high rural figures of this period confirm that the servant population of Aberdeen was a society in which unmarried sexual activity was not unusual. As in the adjacent rural areas premarital conceptions in Aberdeen were frequent. A quarter of first conceptions took place out of wedlock.[8]

The eighteenth century picture of Aberdeen is of illegitimacy under 5 per cent of births and usually under 3 per cent (see Figure 5.1). But doubt about the completeness of the record must prevail. As described in Chapter 2, in 1775 the session and the magistrates set up a system by which the alleged fathers of illegitimate children compounded with the church treasurer for a suitable fine for the support of the poor and remained anonymous in the record. Already those marrying irregularly were registering these marriages with the magistrate and paying him a fine. The next year the session admitted that its officers 'were not sufficiently alert' in tracing offenders and decided to transfer the task to one of the town's serjeants. A bigamy case in October 1778 showed that Alexander Morison had not only his 'current' wife living in the city but that his original wife was also present; clearly, tracing of delinquents was failing. So though the series of information continues and the session investigates cases up to 1785, the record will not stand up to quantification.

An urban parish where the tone of the record encourages belief in the thoroughness of the session's investigations well into the eighteenth century is South Leith (see Figure 5.1). The 'fall' in illegitimacy in the 1690s is implausible: it was a period of war, with many soldiers in the neighbourhood, and soldiers then made up 21 per cent of the men named as fathers of the children born out of wedlock. The likely explanation of the drop in the figures is the dispute, at times violent, between episcopacy and presbytery which raged in this parish. In the period 1661–1710 the percentage of first conceptions out of wedlock appears to have ranged between 18 and 44, and most decades was over 30. Clearly, illegitimacy in South Leith was much higher than in the rural neighbourhood.

One other truly urban parish that provides consecutive figures for several decades

Sin in the City

is Edinburgh's Trinity College between 1661 and 1720. Figure 5.2 shows fairly high illegitimacy ratios in the seventeenth century, levels similar to those of Aberdeen, often over 10 per cent, down to 9 per cent for the 1700s and approximately 5 per cent for the 1720s. The level of out of wedlock first conceptions is high, over half the first births in the 1660s and still as high as a fifth in the 1710s. Rural Lothians illegitimacy ranged between 2 and 3.5 per cent in these decades, so we can see that young persons moving into the city for work experienced a considerable change in sexual habits.

As shown in Figure 5.2, Old Machar parish, that is Old Aberdeen, appears to have had an illegitimacy ratio of over 10 per cent in the late seventeenth century and of first conceptions out of wedlock over 40 per cent. In the 1710s the illegitimacy ratio was still over 8 per cent on our figures. There was then a sudden drop to under half that level in the 1720s and onwards. This drop is most unlikely to be real; that the level continued low merely indicates that, once the kirk session lost its grip, it never regained it.

A more sustained grip is seen in the relatively rural suburban parishes of Glasgow and Edinburgh. As shown in Figure 5.4, Glasgow Barony appears to have had an illegitimacy ratio of between 1.7 and 3.2 per cent until 1750, when it rose. Even so, assuming a birth rate of 36 per thousand, illegitimacy stayed under 4 per cent in the 1750s and 1760s, and first conceptions out of wedlock stood under 20 per cent. Govan, still rural at this time, gives similar low levels of illegitimacy, between 2 and 3.5 per cent, in the years 1711–70, and similarly low figures for first conceptions out of wedlock. St Cuthbert's, Edinburgh has less convincing figures. On a birth rate of 36, appropriate for a rural parish, illegitimacy lay between 5.3 per cent and 3.4 per cent between 1661 and 1710. After that the figures fall very sharply below 2 per cent, and a drop of this sort is not credible.

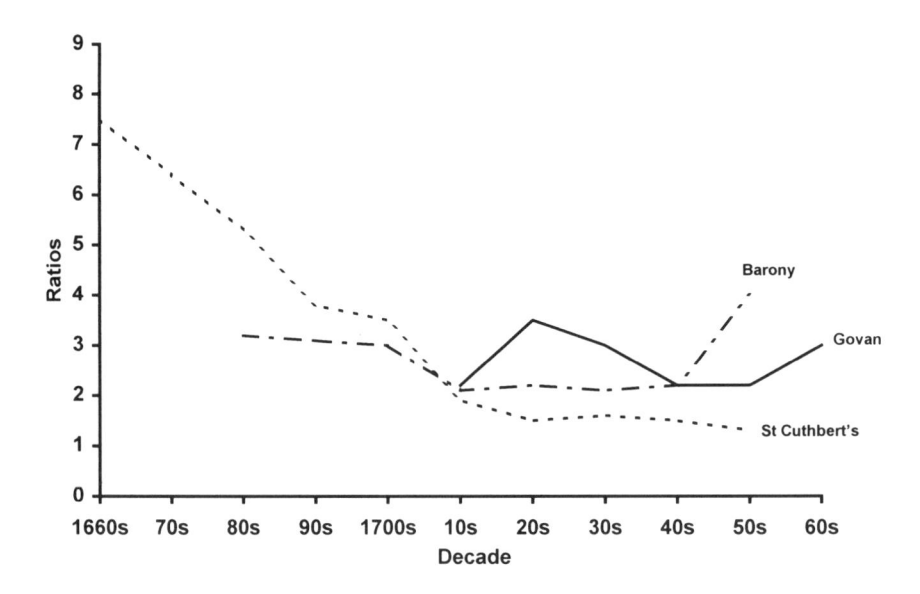

Figure 5.4: Illegitimacy ratios: Govan, Barony and St Cuthbert's

5: Illegitimacy and Bridal Pregnancy

It seems that only in Dundee was urban illegitimacy kept low. In Aberdeen and Old Aberdeen it was higher in the late seventeenth century than the fairly high level of the rural hinterland. In South Leith and Trinity College, Edinburgh, it was markedly higher than in the rural neighbourhood. In the suburban parishes illegitimacy remained low so long as they remained rural, and as they became urbanised the record does not sustain investigation.

In Dundee a consistently high proportion of unmarried conceptions led to bridal pregnancy, as shown in Figure 5.3. In most decades it stood at well over 30 per cent. These figures of high bridal pregnancy continue into the 1770s. In the other city parishes the figure was usually around 20 per cent, and in most the recorded level fell sharply in the early eighteenth century. For instance, in Aberdeen in the 1690s the figure for unmarried pregnancies which brought forth a child within marriage ('antenuptial uncleanness' was the Church's phrase) was about 22 per cent in the 1690s decade; it had fallen to 13.5 per cent in the 1700s and in the 1730s was in single figures. It is unlikely that this fall represents a real change. No characteristic feature of the pattern of marriage, which was the result of a complicated interplay of economic and social factors, was likely to change so sharply. In Old Aberdeen the percentage similarly fell from 26.8 per cent in the first decade of the eighteenth century to 6.7 per cent in the second, another obvious area for scepticism, but it picked up again to over 20 per cent after 1703. Similarly, a sharp drop in St Cuthbert's from 21.5 per cent in the 1730s to 4.8 per cent in the 1740s must reflect both weakening discipline and the ready availability of irregular marriage. The levels of 20–30 per cent which obtained in the seventeenth century, when we have confidence in our figures, show a rough similarity to those found in our earlier study for rural Scotland in the Lothians, and in Aberdeenshire in the eighteenth century. In Dundee the consistently higher figure resembles that of rural Fife.

Another set of interesting figures are those of 'repeaters'. These cases of second or more unmarried pregnancies were labelled successively 'relapse', 'trilapse', 'quadrilapse' or 'multilapse'; the penalties were six appearances for relapse, 26 for trilapse and 39 for anything higher. The proportion of repeat cases falls off during the eighteenth century except in Dundee and Old Aberdeen. In South Leith, for instance, there were 12 repeater cases in the 1690s (14 per cent of the total illegitimate births), 19 in the 1700s (15 per cent), 18 (22.5 per cent) in the 1710s but only three (6.5 per cent) in the 1740s. In the 1750s none were noted, a fact which more probably reflects failure to investigate on the part of the session than successful reformation of male sinners. In Aberdeen only in two decades of the eighteenth century did the percentage of repeater cases get to double figures, and no repeater cases at all were noted for the 1770s. This is not surprising for in that decade the session stopped recording the names of those male offenders who were prepared to pay a stiff fine to the poor's fund. In Edinburgh St Cuthbert's the proportion of repeaters fell off in the 1740s, in Glasgow Barony in the 1760s. Only in Dundee and Old Aberdeen does there appear to have been adequate recording of this feature in the later decades and for Dundee we can find some males with conveniently unusual names in the 1760s who were clearly liberal repeaters and about whom the session was either deliberately or accidentally silent. A relatively high proportion of the cases noted in the later eighteenth century were ones of sustained cohabitation, where it would have been difficult for the session to be unaware of the repeat element. Table 5.2 gives the percentage of cases stated as involving a repeater.

Sin in the City

Table 5.2: Percentage of total cases which involved repeaters

1660s	10.8
1670s	13.5
1680s	16.1
1690s	14.1
1700s	13.7
1710s	12.8
1720s	14.6
1730s	10.4
1740s	9.5
1750s	8.1
1760s	8.2
1770s	7.1

Of both sexes, are men who have extramarital sex more or less likely to repeat the offence as women? (Professional prostitutes do not enter into our sample because, as noted in Chapter 2, the Church regarded them as 'not proper objects of discipline'.) Less effort was certainly put into tracing the past record of male sinners than of women. In Aberdeen, where the justice court handled the same type of case as the kirk session, it is quite clear that the man noted as Mr Thomas Forbes, a gentleman (by the use of 'Mr') and a relapse offender in 1669 with Margaret Robertson is the same man coupled with Margaret Browne in 1672 and not labelled as a trilapse. In the town which recorded the highest level of female relapses, Old Aberdeen, Isabel Scroggie ran as high as a fivefold offender in the 1720s with two of the offences apparently occurring elsewhere. John Miln is noted with her as offender for two of the episodes, but it does not seem to have been a long term cohabitation for her third offence was with someone else.

The explanation for this relatively lax approach is probably twofold. A considerable number of male offenders were people of status: landowners, professional men, merchants, captains of ships, army officers, and in Aberdeen University professors. From these it was unlikely that the session would extract appearances; acknowledgement and monetary support for the child was all that a session could realistically hope for. And the tariff of offences, though comforting to the righteous, made it unlikely that even men of humbler status would go through with the full requirements for instance of absolution for trilapse. It was difficult to get men to the pillar for even single offences; imposing the full tariff would probably meet with total refusal. And this would be bad for the prestige of the Church, besides leaving sinners unreconciled and children unsupported.[9]

If we have to accept that inadequate attention was paid to tracing the past offences of male sinners, the question must remain, how complete is the record of female repeating. We have not found sessions failing to note that a particular woman had been before them before, nor do we find an overstatement of repeat offences. But sessions may, by neglecting some first offences, understate the proportion of repeats. Taking all our parishes together the number of male cases relative to female falls off early in the eighteenth century. Male cases are never as many as a third of the female

5: Illegitimacy and Bridal Pregnancy

in any decade after 1720 and only in the 1660s and 1670s are their numbers approximately half the female. As we do not believe that there was a drastic change in the sexual mores of men in this period we explain our figures by a combination of poor record keeping and increasing readiness to accept double standards. The fall in the level of repeaters, shown in Table 5.2, is probably the result of failure in tracing and identification.

There is no reason to believe that the 'same man' repeater cases indicate a common custom of unmarried cohabitation. If a session used its records to ascertain that a woman was a repeater it would be natural for it to note if the man named was the same or not. In the great bulk of cases the session does not record that the offending male was the same. In Old Aberdeen, for instance, in the 1760s only one of the nine repeater cases was with the same man and there were none in the twenty cases noted in the next two decades. Although Dundee recorded a more steady level of two or three 'same man' repeater cases in each decade we have no reason to suppose that there was a generally accepted folk custom of unmarried cohabitation. Indeed, as will be seen in Chapter 8, the session would assume that such couples had been irregularly married and would demand a marriage certificate. Where unmarried cohabitation did occur it was easy for the session to interrogate the right man, and difficult for him to deny involvement, so the small figures we have for this set-up are disproportionately reliable.

It is dangerous to make positive statements based on figures which are, for the most part, incomplete. Whereas in our study of rural regions we claimed confidence in our quantitative evidence for illegitimacy and bridal pregnancy, we claim no such confidence with regard to any figures presented in this study. However, if we are unable to find out as much as we would like to know about illegitimacy, the material presented in this chapter certainly bears out what earlier chapters have already suggested and what later chapters will underline: that the disciplinary system of the Church failed markedly earlier in the cities than in rural and small town Scotland. Since the efficacy of discipline depended on its universal success, with sinners who ran away being traced and investigated even in distant parishes, the urban failure is probably an important element in the Church's abandonment of the full rigour of discipline in the 1780s.

Notes

Edinburgh, Canongate and Leith kirk session registers are in the Scottish Record Office; the only exception is Edinburgh New Kirk which for the year 1706 is in Edinburgh University Library and for several other years in Edinburgh City Archive. Aberdeen St Nicholas registers are in Aberdeen City Archive; Old Machar registers are in the parish church, with access via Aberdeen University – microfilms of both sessions' records are in the Scottish Record Office. Glasgow Barony and Govan session registers are in Glasgow City Archive, and have not been microfilmed. Dundee registers are in Dundee City Archive, with microfilms in Edinburgh. We have not given references for each citation but always state the month and year, making it possible for anyone to find a particular case.

1 Richard Adair, 'Two Englands? Regional variation in Bastardy and Courtship 1538–1700', in R.M. Smith (ed.), *Regional and Spatial Demographic Patterns in the Past* (forthcoming).

Sin in the City

2   For Webster's census, see J.G. Kyd, *Scottish Population Statistics* (Scottish History Society, Edinburgh, 1952). John Sinclair (ed.), *The Statistical Account of Scotland* 21 volumes (Edinburgh, 1791–7). South Leith catechising lists, SRO.CH2/716/327–8.
3   Rosalind Mitchison, 'Webster Revisited: a Re-examination of the 1755 census', in T.M. Devine (ed.), *Improvement and Enlightenment* (Edinburgh, 1989).
4   Rosalind Mitchison and Leah Leneman, *Girls in Trouble: Sexuality and Social Control in Rural Scotland 1660–1780* (Edinburgh, 1998).
5   A husband did have recourse to the commissary court to prove that a child born during his absence was a bastard and therefore not entitled to the rights of a lawful child, but it was only the propertied who had the motivation to make use of this legal action.
6   The Kilmarnock Old Parish Register gives births by their parity in terms of the father, but it also distinguishes between first and second marriages. It is therefore easy to count the number of births to each marriage, and the average is four.
7   Callum G. Brown, 'The Costs of Pew-renting: Church Management, Church going and Social Class in Nineteenth-Century Glasgow', *Journal of Ecclesiastical History* 1987, pp. 347–61.
8   Gordon Russell DesBrisay, 'Authority and Discipline in Aberdeen 1650–1700' (unpublished Ph.D. thesis, St Andrews University, 1989).
9   The ability of the Scottish Church to bring home responsibility to male offenders compares well with the Prussian state in the city of Neuchâtel, where in the eighteenth century 19 men were convicted of illicit sexual activity and 124 women. A further interesting feature of this city's experience is that in 1755 the state abolished the humiliating practice of public penance and it is after this that there was a marked rise in cases of illegitimacy. Jeffrey R. Watt, *The Making of Modern Marriage – Matrimonial Control and the Rise of Sentiment in Neuchâtel, 1550–1800* (Ithaca and London, 1992), p. 178.

Appendix 2

List of kirk session registers used for our study

Edinburgh:
St Cuthbert's	1661–70, 1681–5, 1692–1756, 1761–80 (+ 1781–90)
Trinity College	1661–81, 1688–98, 1701–3, 1705–6, 1709–22, 1725–7
Canongate	1661–7, 1731–49, 1751–6
Tron	1723–4, 1728–30
New Kirk	1704, 1706, 1709–19, 1735–40
Old Kirk	1707
Old Greyfriars	1711–20, 1732–5
New Greyfriars	1724–8
Lady Yester's	1702

Leith:
South Leith	1661–1780 (+ 1781–90)
North Leith	1697–1700, 1721–80

Aberdeen:
St Nicholas	1661–93, 1701–80 (+ 1781–90)
Old Machar	1674–1760

Glasgow:
Barony	1681–6, 1701–33, 1738–80 (+ 1781–90)
Govan	1711–80 (+ 1781–90)

Dundee:
Dundee	1683–1780 (+ 1781–1800)

6

Evading and Defying Discipline

In our period the majority of Scots, urban dwellers as well as rural, accepted church discipline. There was a small number of individuals in cities who were considered 'not a fit object of discipline' and were therefore expelled the town and not expected to undergo public appearances and rebuke. There was in addition a minority who were considered full members of the congregation but who did their best to evade or defy the control of the Church.

Kirk sessions certainly went to a lot of trouble to trace recalcitrant individuals. The information network whereby a session learned of unmarried pregnant women and other sinners stretched far beyond the bounds of any one parish. In the eighteenth century there developed a highly efficient postal system, and probably no one used it more than kirk sessions. At any given moment in time there would have been numerous letters winging their way from ministers to other ministers, requesting information and assistance. Sessions rarely took any statements on trust but demanded verification.

In Aberdeen (May 1766) Isobel Ross produced a letter from Thomas Cuthbert, the man she named as father of her child, in which he acknowledged this, but 'no member of the session knowing whether the said letter was genuine, the Clerk was appointed to write to the Minister of Brechin where he is said to reside'. The Brechin minister advised the session that Cuthbert had acknowledged writing and signing the letter. Eight years later (September 1774) Aberdeen session similarly insisted on writing to the minister at Kemnay parish in spite of Barbara Thomson's production of a letter from Duncan Carmichael acknowledging guilt; again the minister there was able to reassure the session that the letter was genuine.

However, scepticism was often warranted. Agness Gentleman in Trinity College (December 1703), needing the acknowledgement of her seaman lover to be admitted to penance, forged a letter from him admitting guilt, and claimed that it had come to her in the post. But 'the said letter having nothing of the post Mark on the Back thereof' the ruse failed. Margaret Lamen came before Dundee session in September 1768 and named David Bruce, sailor, as father of the child she had borne four weeks earlier. The session learned that there had been no one by the name of Bruce on board the ship she had named; furthermore, all the hands on that particular ship had been paid off and had left the parish at the beginning of October, '& consequently the child behoved to be three months old in place of one if it had been to such a Man as she gives out for the Father of it.' Grizel McLarin in North Leith (May 1749) was determined to avoid appearing as an adulteress, insisting that she had a letter attesting to the death of her husband, Henry Buchan, although she did 'not know what became' of it. After continual pressure by the session, in March 1750 she finally produced a letter dated 6 January 1748, which she claimed to have got 'from a sailor at Borrowstounness but knows not his Name'. The letter gave 'account of her

6: Evading and Defying Discipline

husband's being lost att Portsmouth Rocks in ship wreck', but the session, informed 'that there was no such man in the ship the Grayhound as Henry Buchan', reckoned the letter a forgery.

In one instance a session's reliance on the post ran into difficulties. Old Aberdeen session (September 1750) wrote to the minister of Banff regarding James Elder, alleged father of Margaret Christie's child, but Elder was postmaster there, and the session, receiving no reply to its letters, suspected that he was intercepting them. It was decided to send a letter via a different system (the 'North Post'), which had the desired effect of bringing Elder to a confession.

Ministers from all over Scotland congregated in Edinburgh every year for the General Assembly, and after such an occasion (August 1704) one of the Aberdeen ministers made enquiries about Margaret Deans, who had been found in bed with John Mowat before she went south. Mowat denied carnal dealing, and the minister's brief was to find out if she was pregnant. He was able to inform his session that some 'honest women in the same house' as Margaret told him that she was not with child.

Attempting to trace women rumoured to have left the parish while 'with child' could take up a good deal of sessions' time. (It is our impression that sessions were more assiduous in attempting to trace such women than to trace men named as fathers, but this is not quantifiable.) In July 1743 Aberdeen session heard that Marjory Kempt was in Banff and wrote to the minister there; the latter replied that she was with her sister in Forglen, so the session wrote there. However, in October it was rumoured that she had brought forth a child in Leith, so a letter was sent to the minister there, who, in January 1744 advised the session that she had not been found. In October 1748 Aberdeen session wrote to the minister of Glenbervie parish regarding Christen Anderson, and that letter crossed one from that parish in which the minister had written that a stranger woman had lately borne a child; she claimed to be married to a sailor, but he was suspicious and wondered if a woman had absconded from Aberdeen. It was indeed the same woman, and she eventually returned to satisfy discipline in Aberdeen.

Thus, in spite of the system of testificates, and the information network, some individuals did attempt to evade discipline by fleeing. In some cases it was simply noted that the sinner had fled. In approximately two thirds of these cases the person fleeing was a woman. This was not a common course of action: just under 4 per cent of women under investigation took this action. There were many practical difficulties in the way of abandoning service and finding support in another parish, and anonymity was difficult. Indeed, most of the women who fled either returned or were traced. There were other methods of escape, more available for men than for women. Men could, for instance, join the army. In all towns, but particularly in ports, there were activities which legitimately called for absence; seamen, merchants, carters, the servants of the upper class who had gone to their estates, all had good reason to be not available. It was relatively easy for a session to pursue someone in a neighbouring parish, and we have not counted such cases as 'gone away'. For example, a noticeable number of Govan's cases involved Glasgow merchants. Absence could be involuntary: William Blackwood, flesher in Govan in 1745 was 'taken prisoner by the rebels' at the battle of Falkirk. All together, some 15 per cent of men managed either temporarily or permanently to be not available for discipline. Women who did so were much fewer, about a sixth of the number of men.[1] But for both sexes the persistence of the sessions usually ended in admission of guilt either

Sin in the City

in person or by letter.

For a time one session, Aberdeen, had many more sinners fleeing. Between 1661 and 1700, out of 543 cases, 63 women and 24 men were reported to have fled. This was probably the result of the drastic penalties imposed by the secular Justice Court. Those who did not pay their fines were subject to a public flogging. When the Justice Court relaxed its severity in the eighteenth century the numbers fleeing fell sharply.[2]

The trouble with fleeing was that sessions had exceedingly long memories, and anyone eventually returning home would still have to satisfy discipline. George Keith fled Old Aberdeen after confessing to fornication in June 1708 and was declared fugitive; he returned in November 1713 and had to make his public appearances. James Clayton, 'mariner', accused of adultery in June 1708, appeared before Dundee session in February 1710, 'and being informed... that he behoved to compear in Sackcloth he went to the Mark door as he sayd to mak water & drew the barr and escaped and hid himself and no accompt could be got of him.' But when Clayton returned home from sea in November 1712 he was forced to make his public appearances, in sackcloth.

If fleeing was a less than ideal way of evading church discipline, were there others more successful? One sure way was to be a member of another 'communion'. The likelihood of this was greatest in Aberdeen, where Catholics and Quakers, taken together, comprised up to 10 per cent of the population in the second half of the seventeenth century. Gordon DesBrisay commented that they posed a threat to the 'unity and cohesion which played so integral a part in the life of the early modern urban community'. The years between 1660 and 1680, he wrote, 'witnessed an unprecedented degree of religious persecution in Aberdeen'.[3]

However, when John Cowie confessed to fornication with Christian Steiven in February 1686, he did so to the minister rather than session because he was a Quaker, and it was recorded only that he asked for a delay in appearing as he was going out of town. Quakers continued to surface in eighteenth century minutes, but neither Aberdeen nor Old Machar (Old Aberdeen) session attempted to exert control over them. For example, in the former parish Mary Elmslie, a Quaker, was reported to be with child to William Keith (April 1722); Keith confessed and satisfied discipline, but Mary was not even cited. Similarly, in the latter parish William Troup confessed to antenuptial fornication with his wife, Christian Mercer; she, as a Quaker, was not called upon either to appear before the session or to satisfy discipline.

There was at least one Quaker family in Glasgow Govan parish as well. In May 1720 William Purdon confessed to antenuptial fornication with a woman he had married irregularly, and also to paternity of an illegitimate child born to another woman, but the session did not feel able to proceed in his case because his father was a Quaker and he had therefore never been baptised. In April 1733 Jean Haddine finally confessed that the true father of her child was not an unknown assailant as she had first claimed, but John Purdon, a Quaker, who 'swore her not to discover him'. The session cited him, but he 'Declined to obey their Appointments in Regard that he was not of their Communion'.

The attitude of sessions to Roman Catholics was far harsher, although when Robert Collisone was named as father of her child by Jean Fraser in August 1673 it was reported that he had confessed privately to the minister, 'but being papyst could not give satisfaction to the session', which suggests simple acceptance of the fact.

6: Evading and Defying Discipline

Roman Catholics continued to come before both Aberdeen sessions throughout the eighteenth century. In February 1703 Old Aberdeen asked the presbytery's advice regarding James Nicol, who had confessed to fornication with Margaret Miln, 'he being popish'. The difficulty was resolved a year later when he renounced 'the popish faith' before the magistrates. Since the purpose of penance and appearance was the re-entry of the sinner to the religious community this could not be offered to those of a different faith. The strength of feeling against Catholics certainly comes across in a case of irregular marriage in Aberdeen in June 1706. The adherence of David George and Margaret Burnet was taken before the session, but at the same time:

> The session did also lay before them the sinfulness and scandal of their Marriage, as being persons of a different Religion, he a profest papist, and she a profest protestant, and shewed the contrariety thereof to the express will of God revealed in his word, did rebuke them sharply, and exhorted them to unfeigned Repentance, particularly the said Margaret Burnet was seriously Exhorted to consider the offence given to God in marrying with ane Idolater (such as all papists are) and the scandal she has thereby given to the Church of God, and the dreadfull snare and temptation to apostasie she hath thereby exposed herself to.

Intimation was to be made from both pulpits the following Sunday, 'that all may know how sinfull such unequal marriages are and avoid them for the future.'[4]

When James Elphinston of Wattle confessed fornication 'privately' to the magistrates of Aberdeen in May 1707, the session asked them to oblige him to appear before the session. He did so in June, and the session regretted having to leave him unabsolved, the moderator exhorting him to 'renounce the popish Religion, and come to our Communion.'

Aberdeen was not the only city to have Roman Catholics. Edinburgh Trinity College session asked the presbytery what to do about Claud Muirhead, a Roman Catholic fornicator, in January 1666 and was advised to speak to the civil magistrate about him. In the same parish in December 1687 Margaret Paris and Patrick Drummond, guilty of a relapse in fornication together, reportedly 'profess themselves to be papists'. In South Leith, in August 1711, Captain Bernardo Delaguardo, a Spaniard, was accused of cohabiting with Janet Hendry, who had fled. He denied the charge (a shipmaster 'having interpret his Language'), but witnesses declared seeing them in bed together and hearing them own one another as man and wife. The session, 'considering that he is a roman catholick and a foreigner referrs him to the magistrats for the execution of the law'.

Thomas Baxter's unsuccessful attempt at evading discipline in North Leith (March 1713) was breathtaking in its audacity. He gave the session a signed declaration acknowledging his fall in fornication and that he now

> thought himself bound in Conscience to be received into the bosom of the Church of England after so foul a transgression, and produced an Absolution from one who pretended to be a Minister of that Church, dated at Edinburgh and (contrary to the present established order of this national Church) declines the Presbytery's Jurisdiction and obstinately refuses to submit to discipline for removing the scandal in an orderly manner notwithstanding of his having lived in the communion of this Church till that time.

Sin in the City

He was to remain under the scandal and be debarred from church ordinances.

As noted in earlier chapters, the second half of the eighteenth century saw the development of schism within presbyterianism. In Dundee and Glasgow in particular, anyone disaffected with the established church had a choice of other presbyterian congregations to join. In Dundee Catharine Macknab gave birth to a child in July 1768 but ignored citations; in September she sent word that 'she would not compear before the session she not being of their Communion'. The session would have had every confidence that she was being disciplined by the minister of her own congregation. The co-operation between denominations can be seen when Peter Ferguson confessed to Glasgow Barony session in September 1789 that he was the father of Jean Boyd's child, 'and at the same time declared that he is a member of the Relief Congregation at Anderston.' The session appointed that 'information of this to be given' to the minister of that congregation.

But what of that much longer established Scottish church, the Episcopal? In Edinburgh Old Greyfriars parish (August 1715) the man named as father of Margaret Mitchell's child, William Monteith, 'Writer', refused to appear before the session, 'on Account that he is not of the Communion of this Established Church'. The father of Catharine Graham's child in Edinburgh New Greyfriars parish (September 1724) was alleged to be Archbald More, brother to the Laird of Leckie in Gargunnock parish. The latter session replied to New Greyfriars' letter by advising that More acknowledged his guilt 'but told he was none of our Communion And therefore could not compear before our Judicatorys.' St Ninians session (August 1740) replied to a letter from Canongate session regarding John Glass of Lachy, the alleged father of Isobell Jois's child, stating that he acknowledged guilt, 'but he not being of the Communion of the established Church refused to submitt to the Censure thereof.' The designations of these three men are very revealing, for after 1690 the Episcopal church became largely a church of the gentry. If one wished to evade the discipline of the Church of Scotland, it was certainly helpful to be able to claim gentility.

In South Leith in February 1692 it was reported that 'my lord Mortune hath incarcerat Mary McIntosh in the tolbuith of Edr becaus she would father the child upon his lordship'.[5] This level of power – or, rather, abuse of power – was atypical in our period, but the ideal of all men and women being equal in the eyes of God was hard to sustain in a hierarchical world. Edinburgh's Trinity College parish had a high proportion of gentry visitors and residents, and various seventeenth-century cases show the session absolving them without demanding public appearances. For example, there was Mr George Fortoun, Chamberlain to Lord St Clare and Bailie of the Regality of Dysart, who in April 1685, 'upon weighty considerations was absolved'.[6] During the episcopal period bishops could be used to get at gentry sinners who might listen to admonitions from members of their own class when they would ignore presbyteries.

Edinburgh New Kirk session had to deal with Mr Charles Menzies, Writer to the Signet, whom Janet Robertsone had accused in October 1712 of fathering her child. He paid for the upkeep of the child after its birth but ignored the session's citations. In April 1713 a committee was formed to 'discourse Mr Charles Menzies... anent his submitting to Church Discipline', but it had to report that Mr Menzies had signified his 'aversion' to attending the session. The session continued chasing him, but in February 1714 it was reported that Menzies was 'obliged to abscond and goe out of the way by reason of his bad circumstances.' Another 'writer' in New Kirk parish, Robert Dalrymple Junior, confessed to fornication in September 1737, but 'refused to appear in publick in order to remove the scandal'. Mr James Gordon of Carnbrogie, who confessed to a committee from Old Aberdeen session that he was guilty of fornication with Barbara Hill (October 1739) did not entirely get off public appearances, but he was allowed to sit in his own seat while he received a single rebuke before being absolved, 'upon paying something considerable to the poor.'[7]

The father of Anne Roy's child was Mr James Nisbet, chaplain to my Lady Lundie. The case came before North Leith session in November 1718, though at that time she lied about the true father. As she had only recently arrived in the parish the session decided that she should satisfy discipline in Edinburgh Old Kirk parish where she came from, but as the scandal had not broken out till she arrived in Leith, Old Kirk session sent her back. When the true father's name emerged, the presbytery was asked where public appearances should be made and decided that 'because of Prudential considerations' it would be 'most of the Interests of Religion' that North Leith should do the censuring. So, although Nisbet had to appear before the congregation, it was a congregation of people who did not know him.

Edinburgh St Cuthbert's session did try to bring Sir Robert Baird of Saughtonhall to heel but caved in at the end. In April 1716 the moderator advised the session that Sir Robert could not deny his guilt with two different women, 'but he refuses to compear publickly before the Congregation, but is content to pay the pecunial mulct for these Enormities. After which the session declared their resolution to proceed against him in a disciplinary way for these crimes.' They ordered their clerk to write to Alloa session, where the women resided, to oblige them to appear here 'in order to give their Judicial confession, that they may have better ground to prosecute the said Sir Robert.' Nearly two years later, in January 1718, a committee reported that Sir Robert judicially acknowledged his guilt: 'he expressed his sorrow for his manifold Iniquities, and particularly for the offence he had given God, and man by his Uncleanness, and solemnly promised thro' Grace henceforward abstinence from all evill, and a thorough reformation of manners and humbly begged the assistance of their prayers to enable him to the performance of what he had promised'. The session approved of this, so much so that they decided that as he 'has in some measure answered Church discipline here' (in spite of never having appeared before the whole session, let alone before the congregation) Alloa session should discipline the two women there.

Not all sessions caved in when it came to members of the gentry. In June 1699 Mr Thomas Gordon, sometime Regent of the College of Glasgow, was named before Old Aberdeen session as the father of Jean Johnston's child. He tried various delaying tactics, eventually appealing from the presbytery to the synod, which dismissed his appeal. He finally confessed his guilt in May 1701 and underwent discipline. But even the most determined and assiduous sessions could be foiled in their attempts to bring members of the gentry under church discipline.

For example, the same Mr Charles Menzies (Writer to the Signet in Edinburgh) who appeared earlier in this chapter was named by Jannet Petrie in Aberdeen in November 1704. (She admitted that she had also been in bed with Mr Moris, fencing master, but he was 'Popish' and therefore referred to the magistrates.) Menzies denied guilt, but after hearing witnesses' depositions the session found 'the scandall is sufficiently proven'. Menzies was ordered to appear publicly but failed to do so.

When asked at the end of May why not he said it was because his oath of purgation was not taken. The session, 'considering the insufficiencie of the forsaid Reason because the session had such gross and clear presumptions of his guilt from the Knowledge of eye witnesses... as that neither their Judicatorie nor any other can admitt of ane oath of purgation' ordered him again to appear publicly. A week later, being asked why he had failed to do so do, he 'gave no answer, only he said that there were some mistakes betwixt the session and him in this process.' The session tried to pin him down, and he eventually admitted guilt but said he had business in Edinburgh and asked for a delay until the end of August, judicially promising to appear then. But at the end of August his brother advised the session that he was too busy to come, and there is no record of him ever appearing in Aberdeen.

Another example was William Grierson of Lag who was reported in August 1708 to have sinned with Elizabeth Arthur. He confessed his guilt to Edinburgh New Kirk session in February 1706 but then employed various delaying tactics to avoid appearing publicly. By September 1710 the session was threatening him with the sentence of lesser excommunication because he had never satisfied discipline, but in November he was elected a Member of Parliament and went to London. It is worth emphasising here that sessions' attempts to get members of the gentry to satisfy discipline, and the latter's attempts to evade this, were not made on pecuniary grounds, for gentlemen usually paid for the upkeep of their illegitimate offspring; it was the humiliation of being compelled by men of lesser rank, let alone stand before a congregation, that was the crux of the matter.

What about female members of the gentry or wealthy families? They received a high degree of protection – both to prevent them indulging in premarital sex and to ensure that the scandal did not become known if they did so – therefore they rarely appear in session records. Aberdeen session tried very hard to enforce discipline in the case of Nicolas Strachan, daughter of Bailie Thomas Strachan. A committee spoke to the bailie in August 1731 and reported that

> about the beginning of January last he was to his very great surprise acquainted by his wife That their daughter Nicolas had aborted of a child sometime in July preceeding, but that she was married to the man who was the father of the child – though in a clandestine and irregular way, and that the man was his own old servant John Gordon, to whom the child was, and who had so married their daughter, and that she her self and others had concealed till then from him, for fear of irritating and provocking him against his daughter, and that she was presently with her mother in the house of Brightmoney in Murray.

He produced no evidence of a marriage, and the session was determined to question her, but Bailie Strachan 'declined' to bring his daughter back home. The session wrote to the minister at Auldearn asking him to cite her before Aberdeen session; he asked for a delay for her on account of her poor health. In December she herself wrote asking for a further delay. After much deliberation the session agreed, because Gordon was abroad at the time but expected back in the summer, and because her relatives promised they would bring her back then 'and shall plead no more delays'. In August her uncle asked for a further delay. In November Gordon's brother advised that Gordon would not be back for some months, and the session agreed to delay the case till the following May. There is a brief gap in the records at that time, but it seems very unlikely that Nicolas ever did appear before the session.

6: Evading and Defying Discipline

North Leith's long pursuit of a male member of the elite, Mr Alexander Ainslie Junior, wine merchant, had a more satisfactory outcome. In April 1720 Janet Marshal, who had been his father's servant, named him as her partner. In response to his citation he wrote that 'his attendance on the Session this day would be the only way to make the business so publick, as soon to arrive at his father's ears, which undoubtedly would do him much prejudice and likeways prove pernicious to himself, and therefore beg'd such favourable measures might be taken, as may prevent the evil Consequences of the affair.' The session, knowing that Ainslie's father really was ill, asked the advice of the presbytery committee for difficult cases and was advised to delay the case 'till the Session see the event of his father's sickness.' His father either recovered or died, for in October Ainslie Junior was cited again though it was reported that 'he declines to appear'. He then went to London on business; on his return he was cited several times but always claimed pressing business elsewhere. In June 1721 he cited 'HM Act of Indemnity of 8 September 1720, particularly paragraphs on pages 29 and 30'.[8] Once again the case was referred to the presbytery committee for difficult cases which advised that he must appear publicly. At last, in February 1722, he began his appearances.

It was not only members of the gentry who used delaying and evasion tactics. In Dundee in June 1706 two couples who had confessed to antenuptial fornication said they would obey the church's discipline providing that two other couples 'who were equallie guiltie of that same sin some years agoe will path the way to them'. Amazingly, the session accepted the justice of this, and though they spent years trying to get the earlier couples to give satisfaction the later couples were allowed to wait until they did. Less successful was the plea of John Macklachlan, periwig maker, before Aberdeen session in March 1716 that he had been absolved by Dr George Gairden, who had officiated 'in the time of the late horrid rebellion'. The session did not think this could be valid but asked the advice of presbytery, which confirmed that any absolution performed by a deposed Episcopal minister was null and void.

Control and discipline of members of the armed forces was in the hands of those forces, not parish ministers. Many men could fall into those categories. In South Leith between 1680 and 1700 over 20 per cent of men named as fathers of illegitimate children were soldiers, and a further 4–5 per cent were sailors. And in the first two decades of the eighteenth century the percentage of soldiers named rose to between 23 and 25 per cent, and of sailors to around 9 per cent. Similarly, Aberdeen in the 1720s had around 20 per cent soldiers (and one sailor), and around 16 per cent and 5 per cent in the 1740s, with the balance shifting to seagoing men in the 1750s with around 18 per cent soldiers and 21 per cent sailors. Thus, while the proportion of sailors varied, soldiers made up about a fifth of men named as fathers of illegitimate children in the above parishes over a long period of time.

Aberdeen session occasionally tried to exercise discipline over such men. For instance, it tried to get John Stewart, a soldier, in October 1717 stationed in Montrose, to appear. A letter from the captain of his regiment advised that Stewart admitted guilt 'but can not be dispensed with for coming to this place and removing the said scandal by reason of the constant use they have for him at duty untill about the middle of February'. In February the session was advised that he still could not be dispensed with, at least until June. In June the regiment was stationed some distance away and about to go abroad, so the session gave up and suspended the

Sin in the City

process against him.

The rise in irregular marriage (chronicled in a later chapter) provided women with opportunities for delay and evasion. In July 1711 Jean Rory was cited before North Leith session for being with child. She declared that she was married to Samuel Lees, soldier, and produced a marriage certificate signed by Mr Crookshanks which the session judged to be forged. She said that she was unable to produce any other evidence, and the session asked the advice of the presbytery committee for difficult cases which suggested writing to the parish where Lees was quartered to see if he adhered to the marriage.[9] In October 1712 the session heard from Mr Crookshanks that he had never married them and that the certificate was definitely forged; Jean insisted that she had got the certificate from Lees and knew nothing about the forgery, but early in 1714 it became known that Lees denied being married to her, and she was to begin appearances for fornication.

However, she disappeared without making her appearances and was found by the minister in the course of visiting families in February 1717. She now claimed to be married to another soldier. She 'Judicially confess'd that a man whom she took to be a minister had formerly married her to Samuel Lees to whom she had a child but seeing the Session was not Satisfyd with the testimonial of that marriage She had not any more owned Samuel Lees as her husband and was married since upon the 21st March 1715 by Mr Thomas Frazer in the Canongate to one William Dawson Souldier in Forfars Regiment to whom she had the Child in her arms'. She produced 'a paper as from Samuel Lees Declareing that he was not married to Jane Rory'. When the session asked 'why she went out of the way, and did not submit to discipline, she said she was never far out of the way but in South Leith but that she had not the will to be Rebuked before the Congregation till Samuel Lees was first Rebuked'. She added that Dawson had been discharged from the army and she did not know where he was. 'Considering the intricacy of the matter', the session referred the case to presbytery.

Another 'intricate' case was that of Isabel Murray, cited for fornication before Edinburgh St Cuthbert's session in January 1736. She claimed that the child was to her husband, Murdoch Mcdonald, and produced a certificate 'which the Session found to be forged'. She was ordered to bring her husband and witnesses to prove the marriage but failed to do so. She managed to spin things out until July 1737 when she produced a letter which she said was from Murdoch McDonald in Uist, 'the missive desiring her to come the Length of Inverness & he would meet her there, for he could not come hither because his Master was adieing'. The session, suspecting her probity, thought 'the Letter was but Shamm & Trick because any Unknown hand might have wrote the Letter'. The minister therefore wrote to the minister at Uist, 'that they may know whether the Letter she produce be a forgery or not'. In December the reply came from South Uist; the minister there 'could find none of that name in all the Countrey & was much of the mind that none of that name was in North Uist either because Murdoch is a name seldome or never used among the Mcdonalds'. It was May 1738 (by which time she had borne a second child) before Isabel admitted that she had never been married.

Delays could also occur when a woman named as father of her child a man who could not be traced. This will be discussed more fully in the next chapter, but one case merits mention here. Janet Jargen first told Glasgow Govan session in November 1760 that her party was 'a Highland Officer that she does not know',

6: Evading and Defying Discipline

which the session did not believe. In January she was pressed to reveal the real father and said that 'she would take a week or two to think upon it and see if she could find out the Man. The session being of opinion that the end of her asking a week or two was only that she might have time to form more Lies further urged her that she should presently declare the truth Answered that it was to Mr Archbald Buchanan, a young man about eighteen years of age who left Glasgow about three months ago and went to Virginia.' She promised to write to him. *Nearly three years later* – in November 1764 –

> the session being fully persuaded that she had hitherto been dissembling and carrying on an obvious Train of Falsehood she was solemnly [exhorted] by the Moderator to be at last ingenuous and declare who was the true father of her child she said she would think upon delating the true father by which every one of the session understood that she departed from accusing Buchanan whom she had formerly mentioned. Being further exhorted and the session expecting she was to make a free confession she said she would tell no more than what she had done before. She acknowledged she had not wrote to Buchanan as she had been appointed but said she intended to do it.

All that the session could do was to refer her to the presbytery.

In another Govan case there was some doubt about the facts, but the attempt to evade discipline entirely did not succeed. In January 1762 John Walker and Margaret Jackson, both married, were accused of adultery. Walker confessed and 'appeared to be very penitent'. Margaret denied 'but in a faint Manner by saying that if it was so she did not know of it and was sleeping or that she thought it was her own Husband.' They were both ordered to begin public appearances, 'to which none of the Parties made any Objection.' However, in February Margaret's husband came to the minister's house

> and spoke about the Matter Alledging that as the Woman was not convicted of Adultery she ought not to be Publickly Rebuked And that she being in a Panick before the session and could not Refuse it in so strong as Manner as she ought what Walker pretended to Confess And that the matter ought to be further examined into before she make any Publick Appearance.

The case was referred to the presbytery for a decision, and in July, 'after long reasoning' it advised thus:

> That both of them be rebuked publickly before the Congregation he as guilty of Adultery according to his own Confession tho there is no Sufficient Evidence of this guilt besides that, as also for his acknowledged drunkenness at that time And she for her acknowledged Drunkenness the Night on which he alledges the said Guilt was Committed.

The chapter so far has been about individuals and groups who evaded, or attempted to evade, the discipline of the church. Out and out defiance is a very different matter.[10] Recalcitrant women are not common in kirk session registers, but they did exist, and there were more of them in towns than in the country. Margaret Harvay, servetrix, was delated to South Leith session by Alexander Air in August 1661, for being alone in her cellar with a man in the night time. In Chaucerian vein, 'being reprovd be the said Alexander, shee bad him and all the constables com kisse her back parts'. Recourse was had to the magistrates, as it was in the case of Jeane Abernethie in Aberdeen, a trilapse in fornication. When she appeared before the session in February 1690 she was 'verie insolent and unrepentant' and refused 'to come before Sessione with the Sackcloath about her'.

In South Leith (October 1672) Janet Morton

> who scandalized [slandered] Catheren Fairfull in calling her witch bird, and being proven by witnesses, was ordained to go to prisson till shee find cautione to appear befor the pulpit to be publicklie rebukit for the same, shee did fine caution to doe so, but still shee refused and shund to make satisfaction as shee was ordained therefor this day she was referd de novo to be put in prisson, and to com the nixt Lords day to be rebukit.

A note was added: 'She cam the 27 day, to be rebukit, but did miscarry her selfe to the minister.'

When Isabell Brown was summoned to Dundee session in July 1776 she did not appear 'but sent word that she had nothing to do with the Session & would not appear therein'. However, application was made to a civil magistrate, and she was brought to the session. Certain women expressed willingness to make public appearances, but not in sackcloth; the additional humiliation of appearing in such a hideous garment was more than they could stomach. Jane Benzie's appearance in sackcloth before Aberdeen congregation was delayed in December 1744 because another woman was starting hers, and there was 'but one Sack Cloth Gown', which seems extraordinary. By the time it was again available she had fled the parish.

We mentioned in Chapter 4 that some women convicted of antenuptial fornication were unwilling to begin their married lives with public humiliation. Margaret Borthwick in North Leith was one such. The session referred her case to the presbytery committee for difficult cases in March 1716; the committee's advice was that her case should be 'narrated before the congregation and she then lie under the scandal and be debarred from sealing ordinances'. John Hill's wife in Dundee (July 1776) insisted that 'the Birth of her Child had been precipitated by a fall down a stair'. On hearing that the midwife had declared that the child was full term Mrs Hill said 'she did not regard what the Midwife said & that the session might give themselves no more trouble about that matter for as she had never received nor intended to receive any Church Privileges from them she did not regard them.'

There were types of behaviour which sessions regarded as recalcitrance which we would look on in a different light. In various parishes at various times women attempted to lessen the humiliation by covering their faces. In June 1719 Dundee session 'enacted that non of them hence forth be allowed to appear upon the pillory with a plaid.' Two in Aberdeen were rebuked in May 1745 'for not discovering their faces when on the pillar'. In July 1713 Christian Callender was asked by North Leith session why during her last public appearance 'she did not open her mouth... when desired to speak out to the edification of the people but turned about her back'. She said that 'the people so gazed upon her, when upon the place of repentance, that she could not open her mouth, but was oblidged to turn about her back.' She was told that 'her offence and miscarriage was very great' and she would be absolved only if she 'carrys as becomes' the following Sabbath. (She did not make an appearance and was left under the scandal.) In South Leith in January 1742 Margaret Davidson 'appeared before the Congregation... & being called, stood up, but so soon as the Rev Mr Stevenson began to speak to her, she clapped down on her seat again, & refused to rise to receive her Rebuke.' When asked at the next session meeting why she had behaved like that 'she alledged she felt trembling, & was not able to stand because the man she gave up for the Father of her child was not named'. The session delayed her further appearances 'till she gave better evidence of her sense of the sin'.

Men were far more likely to be aggressively recalcitrant. The beadle of Trinity College, Edinburgh (July 1703), reported to the session that when he summoned William Robertson, a soldier accused of fornication, Robertson 'was in Bed and swore ane Bloody oath if he had been up he would have runn him through'. Similarly, in South Leith (February 1714) the beadle reported that he had not summoned Lieutenant Alexander Corbat 'being affraid of bodyly harm, in regaird that he had threatened him formerly'.

There were many awkward characters among male parishioners. In Aberdeen George Thomson denied fornication in June 1747, confessed in August 1748, and retracted in September, declaring that he 'neither acknowledges his sin of fornication... nor professes Repentance for it'. In South Leith (June 1767) John Bauld refused 'in a most contumacious & insulting manner to compear or give any Satisfaction'. The minister at Glasgow Govan exhorted Robert Buchanan to repentance in July 1761, 'but in the time of the Exhortation he went away declaring he came not there to be exhorted and examined as a Child and would not return again'. In Glasgow Barony (June 1766) James Mausie denied being either irregularly married or guilty of fornication as alleged by Elisabeth Park:

> after venting himself in many words irreverently before the session instead of answering to the Moderator's queries He turned to Richard Newlands one of the Members of the Session And in a menacing manner said to him, You Mr Newlands, I have heard of you, and I know that you kept a parcel of Bad women and Limmers about your house & sailors and other bad folk, and keeps a baudy house, I know you, and I'll see about you yet, and take care of you.

Also in Barony (January 1779) Robert Letham admitted his guilt but while being admonished he 'behaved with the utmost indecency & contempt of the court & as no impression could be made upon him by any thing that could be said The Session considering this high contempt of their authority agreed to lay him under the sentence of lesser excommunication.'

All of these were cases of men behaving badly before sessions, or to officers sent by sessions, but some waited until their public appearance before acting in ways that raised the ire of the session. In April 1701 the moderator of Edinburgh Trinity College session charged Charles Stirling of Kippendowie 'with dreadful miscarriage in the publick place of Repentance when he compeared before ye Congregation Sabbath last... (Viz.): Laughing, having of fruit, speaking to others, And makeing of water And other miscarriages on the pillar, To the great Dishonour of God and offence of the Congregatione.' In spite of witnesses Kippendowie denied the charge, and it took the session many months – until November – to bring him to a confession. He admitted that

> he did Laugh severall times Also that he did have fruit And also did make his water

Sin in the City

doune upon the people that were benaith him dureing the time of the sermon And professed his sorrow therefore But said his makeing his water was of necessity.

In Old Aberdeen Samuel Larivir ('French silversmith') was absolved after his third public appearance in February 1703, but 'notwithstanding of the profession of his Repentance in the forenoon yet had the Impudence to come back the said day to the publick place of Repentance in the afternoon & in mockery & contempt set himself down there to the Great Dishonour of God, Disturbance of his publick worship & scandal of the whole congregation for which bold and daring presumption' he was referred to the presbytery. The presbytery recommended that the session apply to the magistrates, 'and because this riot & scandal is extraordinary and unexamplyfyed that the said magistrats do signify their detestation & abhorrence of it in his examplary punishment'. He told the magistrates that he had done this because of 'a small wager'. The terrible affront to authority was taken seriously by the civil authorities as well: he was fined fifty pounds Scots and imprisoned. And the man with whom he made the wager had to appear publicly before the congregation.

More typical were men like John Forbes (Aberdeen, May 1707) whose 'garb and behaviour... in the time of his publick appearance was both light and indecent', or John Ross, under clerk to the excise office, who at his first appearance before Edinburgh Old Greyfriars congregation (October 1716) 'was so Undecent and Unbecoming that he thereby gave great offence to the Congregation'. Or Robert Thain (Edinburgh New Greyfriars, September 1726), who appeared publicly twice, but 'instead of giving any Evidence of his sorrow and repentance he rather gave further offence by his light and undecent behaviour in the place of publick Repentance'. Or James Mcfarlane, surgeon apprentice (Aberdeen, August 1740) who appeared 'in so rude and contemptuous a manner' that the minister refused to absolve him.

An odder case was that of Alexander Ogilvie in Aberdeen (December 1731): 'when his name was given up to the Minister in order to his being rebuked, he runn by the other delinquents standing with him upon the pillar and went away in great haste by which insolent carriage he gave no small offense to the congregation.' He told the session that 'he saw no fault in it, but if there was, he was sorry for it.' The session decided that that appearance would not count and he would have to make an extra public appearance, and be rebuked for his carriage as well as the original sin. Informed of this he told the session 'in a huffy and contemptuous manner, that he would think upon it.' The presbytery then advised the session that when he appeared before it, 'observing no signs of repentance with him... and that he had contumaciously refused to give obedience to the session's appointments' he was to lie under the sentence of lesser excommunication, and that 'if he continues obstinately impenitent' the session should proceed with the sentence of greater excommunication, which threatened exclusion from all contact with other members of the congregation. A few weeks later he expressed penitence and the sentence was lifted.

Control was effective over individuals who were concerned, whether for spiritual or temporal reasons, to remain full members of the Church. We cannot begin to estimate how many at any given time in a particular parish chose to be outcasts rather than submit to the authority of the Church, but having collected over 5,000 cases from city parishes we can confidently state that it was never more than a very

6: Evading and Defying Discipline

small proportion of the whole in our period. (Of course, this does not include the 'outcasts', whores and others who were not considered 'proper objects of discipline'.) The majority of parishioners accepted, however reluctantly at times, the rules of the Church.

Only one aspect of acquiescence or evasion of the Church's discipline can be quantified, and so examined comparatively over time, and that is the level of admission by men of responsibility for a pregnancy. In our rural study 66 per cent of named men admitted paternity within a month; in some regions in some decades the level of admission was over 90 per cent. In this study the greater opportunities for absence involved in living in a large town and a port led us to ignore the stipulation of one month. In our total sample 64 per cent of the men admitted the fornication, though some of them attempted to evade responsibility for the child. There were also some who did not appear before the session but admitted guilt by letter, perhaps another 1 or 2 per cent. The total level of admission of guilt was therefore very similar to that in rural Scotland.

But there were interesting differences between the cities. From the limited range of surviving material we see a marked falling off of admissions towards the end of our period. In Dundee the level was 86 per cent in the 1680s, and even in the 1760s and 1770s 49 per cent of men admitted guilt. By contrast the limited amount of material we have for the central Edinburgh parishes shows that by the 1730s admission stood at less than 50 per cent and in suburban St Cuthbert's this was the case from the 1740s onwards. Aberdeen also lost the admission of half its cases by 1740, but in Old Aberdeen discipline was still accepted by three quarters of those named in the 1750s. In Glasgow Barony and Govan well over half admitted guilt in the 1770s. The general picture is of the sustaining of effective acquiescence to discipline by the men concerned in Dundee and in the suburbs of Glasgow, but its relatively early loss in Edinburgh.

There is one final aspect of this subject to be considered before the end of this chapter. Discipline was exercised by groups of men, ministers, elders and deacons, who should have been virtue personified. But, of course, they were human and therefore fallible. Andrew Fowler, maltman, who confessed to fornication with Janet Forbes in Aberdeen (January 1726) was a deacon and collector of the session's funds before being deposed for his sin. Old Aberdeen had a guilty elder, similarly deposed, in October 1736. Jane Fraser declared to Aberdeen session in January 1746 that her child was begotten in adultery, by Mr David Brown, Minister of the Gospel at Belhelvie. He too was deposed. But Glasgow Govan session did not consider such a sin to be a permanent bar. One of its elders, James Rowand, confessed fornication in January 1747 and was deposed at that time. The elders who conferred with him after his second public appearance reported that 'he seemed to be deeply affected with his forsaid sin' (as indeed he might), and about a year and a half later (in October 1748) he was restored to the office of elder.

All of the above cases must have caused a certain amount of glee among parishioners, but they pale beside the case of James Smith, session clerk in Aberdeen. In August 1732 Margaret Strachan, a married woman, confessed adultery with Mr Smith, who fathered her child. She declared that on one occasion 'he obligded [her] to sit down upon her knees upon the grass among the corn and hold up her hands and swear that she should never divulge his guilt with him, for that

Sin in the City

thereby he said she would disgrace herself, and turn him out of his post'. Smith's version of the occasion on which she alleged wrongdoing was very different from hers. He said that he had met with her on his way back from the Old Town and she had demanded charity of him, saying that

> she was a woman subject to the falling sickness, & that she had spent considerably upon Physicians for cures That she had a husband who had left her in a miserable condition & who was a soldier in Orkneys Regiment in Ireland & believed that what Drugs & other Portions of Physick she had got, she could have no more children to him & any man. And thereupon all in an Instant (to Mr Smiths great surprize) took up her cloaths & said to him, If you have any Inclination for a woman you may be satisfied, & fell down on her back in that posture, Which on observing cryed, Fy shame upon you for a Woman that you should prostitute yourself in that manner to any man far less to me who am no Dragoon soldier who would not stick to do wickedness with you. And immediately, while he was yet speaking to that purpose she fell a shivering & into a fitt of Epilepsie as it seemed to him; Whereupon lest any body had discovered him coming off from her in that condition he saw it fitt to take down her cloaths & so left her.

Margaret proved that after the child was born he gave her money; and claimed furthermore that he had also been guilty of scandalous conduct with another woman, Christian Lillie, now dead. Smith, of course, denied this, and said to the session that the presbytery had declared, regarding Margaret Strachan, 'that no stress was to be laid, nor credit to be given to any Declaration she had emitted to his Disadvantage'. But the session told him that he had misunderstood what the presbytery said: 'they had only told Mr Smith that Credit might have been given to his Denials of Guilt with Margaret Strachan if the Presumptions had not been so strong against him'. Witnesses were called concerning Smith's conduct with Christian Lillie. One woman declared that on a July evening she was washing clothes in the loch with some other women 'who told her that Mr Smith and Christian Lillie were together on the other side of the Loch; & bad her go and see what they were adoing'. She had waded across the loch, causing considerable confusion to Smith, though he told the session that all he did when he met with Christian was to converse with her 'about her infirm Mother & her Idiot Sister'. But the presbytery found Smith guilty of adultery with Margaret Strachan and scandalous conduct with Christian Lillie. The moderator told him 'to repent of, and give satisfaction of his said offences':

> To which Mr Smith answered, That as he was conscious of no guilt with the saids persons, so he was fully perswaded that there was no regular prooff nor any presumptions inferring any of the said scandals against him, & therefore he could not in Conscience make any profession or repentance for what he was not guilty of, nor submit to this sentence of the Reverend Presbytery, by which he judged himself grievously wronged.

And so, this chapter on recalcitrance ends with someone who had for years been recording the sins of others.

6: Evading and Defying Discipline

Notes

Edinburgh, Canongate and Leith kirk session registers are in the Scottish Record Office; the only exception is Edinburgh New Kirk which for the year 1706 is in Edinburgh University Library and for several other years in Edinburgh City Archive. Aberdeen St Nicholas registers are in Aberdeen City Archive; Old Machar registers are in the parish church, with access via Aberdeen University – microfilms of both sessions' records are in the Scottish Record Office. Glasgow Barony and Govan session registers are in Glasgow City Archive, and have not been microfilmed. Dundee registers are in Dundee City Archive, with microfilms in Edinburgh. We have not given references for each citation but always state the month and year, making it possible for anyone to find a particular case.

1. The statistics apply to individuals who fled immediately after being cited; many more fled before – or during the course of – public appearances.
2. Gordon Russell DesBrisay, 'Authority and Discipline in Aberdeen 1650–1700' (unpublished Ph.D. thesis, St Andrews University, 1989). The comment about the situation after 1700 comes from our own examination of Justice Court records.
3. Ibid., pp. 325 and 328.
4. Linda Colley in *Britons – The Forging of a Nation* (London, 1992), argues that for much of the eighteenth century Protestantism was a defining characteristic of the British, which helped to bind the three nations together; Catholicism was the 'other' which 'we' were not.
5. As noted in Chapter 1, during this period there were two kirk sessions operating in South Leith; this case appears in the Presbyterian register.
6. Other examples are Robert Douglas in May 1665, Mr Francis Hamilton in October 1674, Mr Robert Monteith in September 1675, and James Carnaigie, sheriff depute of Forfar, in July 1675.
7. Barbara Hill, who had been a servant of Lady Carnbrogie, produced a letter from Carnbrogie 'wherein he calls himself her most Loving & dutiful Husband'. She declared that she was not married to him and that she would have told the minister of her guilt some time ago, but that Carnbrogie 'would not suffer her, carrying her out to Fraserburgh & giving out that she was his wife'. Such behaviour should have earned greater censure rather than concessions.
8. No such statute can be found, and we must assume he made it up.
9. Edinburgh was the only presbytery with a 'committee for difficult cases'. The existence of this committee does seem to have produced a certain amount of laziness in kirk sessions in that city; in any case the least bit out of the ordinary the temptation was to refer it to the committee. The decision to write to the parish where Lees was quartered could easily have been made by the session.
10. Some of the material in this, and the next, section appeared in our paper, 'Acquiescence in and Defiance of Church Discipline in Early-Modern Scotland', *Records of the Scottish Church History Society*, Vol. 25 (1993).

7

Lying to the Session

In the last chapter we saw many examples of individuals attempting to evade or defy church discipline, but there is a sub-category of that subject which requires a chapter of its own. The statistics of male denial of guilt (i.e. intercourse) do not reveal the complexities of sessions' attempts to get at the truth. In rural parishes the majority of cases were straightforward; male threats and bribes and female prevarication were rare. The urban scene was very different. Population mobility, the disparity in social class between women servants and their masters, and arguably a greater sophistication on the part of city dwellers meant that attempts at deception were far more prevalent. As noted earlier, Edinburgh presbytery was the only one in Scotland to have a special committee for 'difficult cases'.

Sessions did not give up easily. James Carse in Glasgow Barony denied guilt with Christine Murray in November 1733; the session continued to put pressure on him in the years that followed, and finally, in November 1743 he confessed. Nor did sessions have to take seriously remarks like that of James Bannerman in Old Aberdeen who in May 1753 declared that 'tho' he were going to the Gallows, he never had any carnal Dealing with her', as he confessed his guilt six weeks later.

Why did men deny responsibility? An obvious reason is finance. George Taylor in Edinburgh St Cuthbert's (May 1745) told a witness that he would not have denied his guilt with Janet Miller 'but that he was in no condition to bring up the Child'. However, a wish to avoid public humiliation, and for married men fear of exposure, appear to have been stronger motives than the financial one.

Masters also exercised social control over their apprentices. Hugh Walker in South Leith (October 1719), 'said that if he should confess he would run the risk of the penaltie of his Indentures, being an Apprentice'.[1] In Edinburgh Trinity College (February 1722) Mungo Campbell's master told an elder that the only reason Campbell denied guilt was 'because if he would Confess the same he knows that by his Indentures he would be obliged to serve him for more years than are therein contained.' In South Leith (April 1725) Jean McDonald declared that the father of her child was her master's apprentice, 'and that his apprenticeship being within two months of running out, he desired her to conceal it as long as possible, that so he might get up his Indentures before it was known'.

Some two to three per cent of men confessed they had been guilty with the woman but denied paternity. For the most part this was doubtless merely an attempt to avoid paying aliment for the child. It is unlikely to have proved successful, for by the later eighteenth century sessions were taking care that the support of illegitimate children should not fall on the parish. However, one should not altogether discount male fears that the child assigned to them was not really theirs. Genuine doubt may have come from an incorrect and over rigid concept of the length of gestation. It was common to assume that gestation took nine calendar months from the day of

7: Lying to the Session

intercourse, a calculation which varies by the season and leaves plenty of opportunity for a child 'not to come to the right time'. In South Leith (January 1726) James Gifford would not own himself to be father of Elizabeth Thomson's child 'unless she would swear that the child was his & then he would take with it.' The session decided he was 'crazy in his judgment'. In Glasgow Govan (May 1734) James Robertson denied being guilty with Janet Shadden but 'added if Janet would declare before the congregation that she was free of all other men that then in that caice he would take with the child, which the session looked upon as ane acknowledgment of guilt'. (Understandably so; but he continued denying.) In Glasgow Barony (July 1751) Thomas Ross refused to admit that he was the father of Agness McAlloy's child unless the session agreed to 'make her Depone that she was not guilty with any other man'. The session judged his demand 'unjust' and refused to grant it.

How could sessions even begin to decide who was telling the truth when a woman accused a man and he denied it? Obviously, we cannot always know why certain stories were believed and others were not. Body language, tone of voice and other criteria not recorded in kirk session registers must have played a part. However, in her discussion of witchcraft trials in Scotland Christina Larner emphasised the importance of 'ill fame' in the Scottish legal system.[2] Far from being expected to consider a specific accusation on its own, courts took into account the reputation of the individual accused, and this played a key part in determining innocence or guilt. Nor surprisingly, then, reputation was also an important consideration in kirk session cases.

In April 1711 Aberdeen session did not believe Margaret Bowerman's accusation of John Runcey, footman to the Laird of Foveran and at that time in London. Two elders reported that 'In their inquireing more narrowly into this woman's conversation [behaviour] were made to understand, that her conversation hath been very loose, and that there is not a more vile and naughty woman in a city or place, than what this Bannerman is'. (The word 'naughty' had far more serious connotations in the early modern period than it does today.) Charles Kirk in Edinburgh New Kirk (January 1714), denying Elizabeth Hamilton's accusation of him, 'told that no regaird ought to be had to her testimony because she is infamous and for proving thereof produced ane extract... containing an account how often the said Elizabeth was committed prisoner to the guaird and sometimes to the Correction house by the Kirk Thesaurer and Constables'. Similarly, James Gray, merchant in Canongate, denying guilt with Margaret Brunton in January 1722, produced 'ane Extract out of the City Guard books of Edinburgh, That the said Margaret had been in the house of correction, and that she has enacted herself to Remove herself from the City and priviledges, never to be seen in the same under pain of being scourged... and Concluded that no assertion of such a [woman] as she was ought to be regairded'.[3]

The unfairness of this dependence on previous character for determining the truth of a woman's accusation is particularly evident in the case of Catharine Waddell in Dundee (March 1737). 'Being found grossly Ignorant and considering what a notorious Vile unclean Wretch she was and now Fathering her Child upon a young man now att London the Session did not think her a proper subject of Church Discipline upon which they thought it Convenient that the magistrates be applyed she be Banished the Town.' A week later the young man, who in fact had not yet departed for London, confessed guilt with her.

When Marion Tenent named John Lind of Gorgy before Edinburgh St Cuthbert's in October 1719 the session was not sure whether to believe his denial in spite of 'being certainly informed that the said Marion is a person of a very bad Character being very naughty in all her conversation being marked in their former Minutes for a person of a Loose behaviour, such as drunkenness & prophaning of the Lord's day'. However, in January, 'considering that the place where she says she was guilty with him is an open Trance, thro' which the family pass to more retired rooms, and it being five [o'clock in the] afternoon in May when the Chaplain's teaching the Children, and he declaring to the said Committee that John Lind is a youth of a sweet discreet conversation', the Session dropped the case against him and allowed Marian to make her public appearances without having established who her partner in guilt actually was.

What about men of bad character? Although men did not sell their bodies, sessions took cognisance of unsavoury reputations. Aberdeen, arguably the most misogynous of sessions, also recorded the harshest words about men. For example, in October 1711 it learned that James Stivenson, a chapman named by Barbara Rancy, was 'a man of such a loose conversation [behaviour] and debauched a practise that he always dishaunts and leaves the place where he commits wickedness, and goes to another, for eviteing [avoiding] all Church discipline.' In May 1714 Aberdeen session was advised by the minister in Queensferry that John Aven, the man named by Isobel Cordiner, 'had fought a duel there with an Englishman, mortally wounded him and was fled the country'. Even if he had appeared before the session it was 'not to be doubted but that he would denie all guilt... even upon oath if required, he being believed and looked upon by all that knowes him to be one of the worst of men.' Of another man, Lues Nisbet (January 1729), it was reported that he was 'debauchedly and raikishly inclined'. In April 1722 Old Aberdeen session was even-handed in its condemnation of Jean Urquhart and the man she accused as the father of her child, William Robertson. The elders reported that 'by all the account they had got about him he's generallie by open voice & common fame repute to be a Man very scandalous in his behaviour & every way naughtie & obscene in his Conversation And with respect to the said Jean Urquhart she is reckoned to be as bad & wicked a woman as he is a wicked & profane a man'.

A bad reputation acted against an individual, but likewise a good one acted in their favour. Aberdeen session in May 1712 was sceptical regarding Janet Smith's accusation of William Bannerman, who had left the parish, as she seemed to 'prevaricate', but enquiry revealed that 'her conversation' since she came to the parish, apart from her fall in fornication, 'hath been blameless', so her story was accepted. Similarly, in September 1719, with regard to Christian Smith's accusation of William Prior, soldier, who was abroad, Aberdeen session, 'understanding that the womans conversation hath been orderly before this snare she hath lately fallen into, and that there is no ground to believe that her guilt is with any other man' allowed her to begin appearances.

The above are cases where a man was absent, but reputation also mattered in denial cases. A gentleman, Mr James Baird Junior, denied guilt with Jean Milne (Edinburgh St Cuthbert's, September 1771), but the deacon told the session that Jean's former mistress gave her a very good character and that the neighbours said 'they had never seen or heard any light or indecent thing about her but that she appeared to them to be a good natured simple girl'. Also in St Cuthbert's (January 1768) William Hay, merchant, denied guilt with Margaret Taylor, who had come from Caithness at Whitsunday, 'and as he began to alledge some things touching her Character in Caithness she produced a regular Testimonial dated about the time she left that place properly attested setting forth that when she left that place her Character was untainted'.[4] Similarly, William Paterson, Writer to the Signet, in Edinburgh New Kirk (February 1715), said he was informed that the woman accusing him, Mary Batees, was 'under a bad fame, and no regard ought to be had to her testimony, Whereupon she produced a sufficient testimonial from the Canongate Session testifying her good behaviour'.[5]

Such attempts at character blackening were far from unique. In view of the importance of reputation or 'fame' it is hardly surprising to find some men doing their best to cast doubt on a woman's integrity. But it rarely availed them anything. John Crawford, weaver, a married man, denied guilt with Janet Martin before Edinburgh St Cuthbert's session in March 1765 and subsequently attempted to prove that she had 'a Light Character'. In September he put forward the names of some witnesses for his exculpation. The session, who did not believe his protestations of innocence, asked what he proposed to prove by the witnesses, and he replied that they could prove she was also guilty with other men. The session told him that though such evidence 'may tend to blacken her Character Yet it cannot any way exculpate him', and declined to hear the witnesses. Crawford appealed against the session's decision to the presbytery, but the presbytery upheld the session.

Similarly, in Aberdeen (November 1768) James Low said he could prove that Rachel Duncan, the woman accusing him, had 'long before a bad Character, and an improper Behaviour'. Rachel was able to produce written attestations of her good behaviour, and a witness who declared that 'she was three years in his Service, and had all that time behaved in a very decent and unexceptionable manner.' The moderator told Low that 'tho there was no full proof of his guilt with the said woman, yet probability was altogether against him, and that all the Evidences he had brought to blacken her character, served not in the least to clear him'. Members of sessions were often well aware that a man was lying to them and were not about to let him make fools of them.

In October 1746 John Clark, 'writer' (i.e. lawyer), alleged before Aberdeen session that Margaret Taylor was 'a common Strumpet and notorious Whore, which, he said, he could easily prove, but afterwards own'd that it is very possible, and he does not doubt but he might have had carnal dealings with her some time or other when he was in drink'. For a man to deny guilt and then later claim that he was drunk at the time and did not therefore remember what had happened was not at all uncommon. For example, Christine Stewart in Glasgow Barony declared in April 1747 that her child was begotten in the fields at Dalmarnock when James Moffat accompanied her home after drinking together in a change house in the Gallowgate. Moffat admitted drinking with her and accompanying her home but denied carnal dealing. The session continued to exert pressure on him, and in October he declared that 'he did not remember if ever he had been guilty with that woman, but own'd he was some what the worse of drink the night he convoyed her to Dalmarnock when she says the child was begot, but thinks he was not so much intoxicate but he would have minded that guilt had he committed it'. The Moderator then asked him, 'if he could say he was positive he never had been guilty with her? but still would give no answer than that he could not remember it'. (He did eventually confess.)

In Dundee (June 1760) David Watson, after insisting that he was not the father of Ann Stuart's child, eventually admitted that she came to his bed one night when he was drunk, and 'that if ever he was guilty with her, it was on that Night... That he could not think he was guilty with her that night, as he was then not really capable'. Captain Archibald Seton in Aberdeen (July 1752) 'Denyed that he is conscious of having ever had any carnal knowledge' of Margaret Duncan

> but that Lodging in the House where she served and taking sometimes a Liberal Glass with his Friend in an Evening the Door of the Room where he sleeps being always kept unlock'd any woman or person might have come into the Bed to him without any previous concert on his part and absolutely refus'd guilt with the said Margaret Duncan to the Best of his knowledge though it is possible he might some night or other when in liquor have been guilty of uncleanness with her and as he will not positively swear he was not so he submitted himself entirely to the session to inflict what Censure they should judge proper in such a Circumstantial Case.

As Captain Seton resided in Udny parish the session wriggled off the hook by referring him to that session, 'to Censure him as they shall see Cause.' In all of the above cases the man was not really lying but denying personal responsibility.

If a man denied carnal dealing with a woman, a session could offer him the opportunity of swearing an 'oath of purgation' before the congregation which would clear him of the scandal. He would be given a copy of the oath to consider first. It was strongly worded – more or less threatening eternal damnation if the swearer lied – and the hope was that perusing this oath would be enough to cause a guilty man to confess. Very occasionally a man was actually allowed to swear the oath, for example in Glasgow Govan Thomas Fleeming denied guilt in November 1732 and was finally allowed to swear the oath of purgation in March 1734. But what is striking is the extreme reluctance of sessions to allow the oath to be sworn. For instance, in March 1730 Isobel Kinnaird ('a poor blind woman' in Old Aberdeen) named Robert Smith, a married man, as father of her child. He admitted being with her on the night in question but denied fornication. In August 1732 he expressed willingness to swear the oath, but in October the session delayed tendering it, 'as they were in no ways satisfied about his honesty'. Sessions did not want individuals to add the serious sin of perjury to the sin already committed.

A striking example of community action in such a case can be found in Dundee in 1683. In June John Bowman, a married man, denied guilt, and in September he declared himself ready to swear the oath,

> at which the woman Margaret Fithie mad such ane clamour & the congregatione mad such ane noyse knowing that the presumptions against him wer so strong viz that the woman had committ fornication with him before his marriage & then he had given hir herbes & given hir money to buy aill to boyle hes herbes of purpose to cause hir pairt with chyld.

Not surprisingly, the minister refused to tender the oath and referred him to the presbytery.

When James Bean, who had denied guilt with Margaret Rowan in February 1768, offered in November to swear the oath, Glasgow Govan session, thinking it 'probable he hath been guilty', told him to 'consider well of the offer he had made'. A week later he still denied, 'but in the Opinion of the session more faintly than before'. He then said that before he swore the oath 'he would first have the Woman's Oath whither she had been guilty with any other but him', but the session would not hear of this.

Kenneth Mackintosh denied guilt with Mary May before Aberdeen session in March 1709. The session did not believe him, but he continued denying. The following January, after he had perused a copy of the oath he said that he could not swear it, 'he having uncovered... her nakedness', a clause in the oath. The session judged him guilty, not being 'concerned in those nice distinctions, which many unclean persons invent'. Also in Aberdeen a member of the gentry, Thomas Burnet of Kirkhill, told the session in May 1717 that he was clear to take the oath but did not consider himself obliged to do so as the session had failed to prove the accusation against him by witnesses so he thought himself assoiled (cleared).

> Unto which it was replyed, that however this reason offered by him might sustain befor a Civill court, in matters purely civill inferring at the most a corporall punishment, yet nowayes can it sustain before an Ecclesiastick court in matters of an higher kind, where the conscience of the person is immediately concerned.

Some men offered to swear the oath in front of the session instead of publicly before the congregation. No session ever allowed this, for the theology stressed the Christian congregation as the agent of discipline. Old Aberdeen session (March 1718) told Charles Hay that 'it was contrary to the practise of this National Church'. John Mackie (Old Aberdeen, April 1759) said that 'if the Presbytery or session would take his oath, he would give it but would not make a fool of himself in public'; he was excommunicated a year later. George Neilson, a married man, told Edinburgh St Cuthbert's session in February 1725 that 'he was content to take the oath of purgation before the session, but not publickly'; this was refused him. The following year (May 1726) Neilson continued to aver that he would swear the oath before the session, and the moderator again told him that if he took it at all 'he behoved to take the same publickly, for the presumptions of his guilt were so strong, that every person who knew the affair, were persuaded of his guilt with Janet Chrystie'. In February 1727 an elder reported that Neilson 'seems more inclin'd to undergoe the Censure of the Lesser Excommunication, than to be purged by Oath in face of the Congregation'. In October 1729 the sentence of lesser excommunication was passed against him.

Were women ever asked to swear the oath of purgation? We found only two instances, both in Old Aberdeen, where this was even suggested. In October 1681 Isobel Bruce named a man who could not be traced, and the bishop advised that she would have to swear publicly that the man she had named was the true father of her child. In October 1683 she expressed willingness to do this, 'but there being ground to suspect that she was guiltie of adulterie and she being ane hard hearted stupid Creature her oath was not taken but got the 1st admonition in order to excommunication'. In October 1709 Margaret Brown named George Forsyth, who had since died; in December she was given a copy of the oath of purgation that she knew no other man but Forsyth. However, in January the midwife declared that while giving birth Margaret had continued to name Forsyth as father, and this was considered sufficient proof for her story to be believed without an oath being sworn.

In cases where paternity was in doubt, sessions routinely used midwives to put pressure on women during childbirth (see Appendix 1). The theory was that a woman giving birth risked her life, and in such circumstances would not endanger her soul by lying. Thomas Hamilton, 'chirugeon', denied guilt with Christian Hamilton before Edinburgh St Cuthbert's session (July 1731). As she had continued to name Hamilton when the midwife refused to assist her until she declared who the true father was, 'the Moderator intreated Mr Hamilton to be Ingenuous, for the Session were perswaded of his guilt with her'. In the case of Isobel Hardie in Aberdeen (June 1708), after the midwife declared that in her pangs she had named James Thom (the man she had first accused) it appeared that she was dying, and the minister was called to her: 'and when he went, he found her indeed in a very bad case, however being able to speak, he posed her with all the seriousness he could, and she still named Thom'. (Isobel recovered; Thom continued to deny but was not believed.) However, this means of establishing paternity could be problematical. Jean Waldie in Edinburgh Old Greyfriars (September 1733) had named William Cumming who denied:

> being interrogate as to her giving up another man as the father of her Child Owned that when in Labour & in Agony she to please her relations that were about her did name another man as the father of her Child but does not remember whom she named.

For the most part, if a man denied guilt, sessions demanded some kind of proof, or 'presumptions', from the woman. If a man fled after being accused this was usually treated as an admission of guilt. For example, Emilia Lawson told South Leith session (June 1721) that when she knew she was pregnant she went to Robert Cowan '& desired him to go along with her to the Minister, & that he promised so to do upon Monday last but by that time was fled off the place & had left his service.' The minister checked with Cowan's master and others and found this to be true. The session considered 'his fleeing from the place upon this occasion as a clear presumption that he takes the guilt upon him'.

Financial provision was seen as another likely indicator of guilt. In June 1776 Florinda Bathune asked Dundee session to allow her to begin public appearances for fornication with John Brown of Glasswell, and 'the Session considering that altho John Brown had never appeared before them either to acknowledge or deny, yet as he has undertaken to maintain the child there is the highest probability of his being the Father thereof'. However, some men insisted that they had given the money for other reasons. Katharine Cruickshanks told Edinburgh Trinity College session (October 1711) that the Laird of Bannockburn, brother to the absent man she alleged as her party, 'gave her Twentie shillings sterling very lately to pay the Chylds quarters', but Bannockburn insisted that 'he gave the said Katherin twentie shillings to be free of the Clamour and that he Denyed he knew anything of his brothers being guilty with her'. William Stewart of Hartwood in Edinburgh New Kirk (February 1718), named as father of Elizabeth Hamilton's child, admitted that he had given money to pay the midwife and to bury the child, and that he had satisfied the kirk treasurer, but 'he in the strongest terms asserted his innocency and that it was meerly from ane over anxiety about his reputation being assured by them that the Child being buried the thing would never come to height'. A year later the moderator 'dealt with him to be ingenuous and not to add sin to sin by concealing the truth any longer since there are such strong presumptions of his guilt', but he still denied.

Dundee session would have none of this. John Mcdonald, dancing master, wrote to the session in November 1779, expressing astonishment at the 'presumption' of Isobell Christie in naming him father of her child. On thinking it over, he wrote, he had decided that 'the quietest method to get rid of such a disagreeable affair would be to provide for the Child which I hereby promised shall not come upon the parish', trusting that the session would not therefore 'lay me under the imputation of Guilt'. The session were satisfied with his conduct 'in engaging to provide for Isobel Christie's child' but found that 'his engaging to provide for this Child & at the same time refusing Guilt does not coincide together' and therefore continued to cite him.

For the most part the kind of 'presumptions' demanded were indications of an intimate relationship, and for this the evidence of fellow servants and neighbours was vital. Not all of the witnesses' statement were of equal value. With regard to Charles Hutcheon, who had gone to London before Mary Calder named him as father, a witness told Aberdeen session (October 1772) that as soon as she knew that Mary was pregnant she reckoned that Hutcheon was responsible, because he was 'a light and frolicksome young man'. The session did not accept this as sufficient evidence. In March 1745 a witness declared to Aberdeen session that George Wilson had told him with regard to Christen Stewart that he 'had girded her up'. Being asked 'what was meant by that Expression', he had to admit that he did not know 'what George Wilson meant thereby', which was not much use. In some cases a witness's testimony could disprove a woman's story. Betty Dunning in Edinburgh St Cuthbert's (January 1772) named Mr Pitcairn, wright, as father of her child, but a fellow servant declared that in her opinion Betty was already with child when she arrived in the parish, 'because a few days thereafter she observed her squeamish and not eating her victuals'. (And indeed the child was born too early to be Pitcairn's.)

Most telling, of course, were sightings of the couple in a compromising situation. A witness declared before Aberdeen session (November 1768) that she had seen Margaret Robertson and the man she named as father of her child 'in Bed together in unseemly shape'. Furthermore, when Margaret accused him, 'he answered in her hearing, that it was too soon to know whether she was with child or not'. Others testified likewise, and the session had no doubts about the man's guilt. A female witness in the case of Isabella Grant and Walter Scott in Edinburgh St Cuthbert's (February 1778) declared that she had shared a bed with Isabella one night and that Walter 'came three several times to the Bedside that Night – That he Clapessed Isabella Grant who was asleep – That he wanted to come into the Bed – but that the declarant prevented him and struck him'. Another witness subsequently declared that 'she has frequently seen him Kissing & Clapping [caressing] her for which the declarant often quarrelled him'. However, she added that 'she never saw any other improper Behaviour betwixt them'. He continued denying; the session eventually decided that 'tho' there is no direct proof to fix the guilt on Walter Scott there are such presumptions against him that they cannot assoilzie him'.

The denials of a married man, William Green, dancing master in Dundee, of guilt with Helen Mackay (May 1776) became less convincing after her landlady declared that 'Wm Green had a Custom of standing before Helen Mackays Windows & when he could not see her he gave half pennies to Boys to call Helen Mackay to him'. Also

Sin in the City

in Dundee (October 1779), a neighbour of Agnes Milln's declared that she knew that Alexander Galloway, who had denied guilt, often visited Agnes and would be told by the servant girl 'that the Sweetheart was there'. Another witness declared that 'she did suspect them of being guilty together that Night as she heard what she thought was not over decent & that she told Agnes Milln pretty sharply about it next day'. In Edinburgh St Cuthbert's (January 1775) James Milligan confessed guilt with Elizabeth Mosman but insisted that it had not happened after February 1774 so he could not be the father of her child. But a witness declared that in the summer, 'happening to go into the Kitchen he found the said Milligan and Mosman toying together in an undecent manner'.

Richard Barton in Dundee denied guilt with Janet Ewing (November 1722), claiming that there was another gentleman who looked very much like him who was the real father, (the only one of our sample who tried a version of the 'identical twin brother' trick). Janet's master and mistress declared that the couple were found on the night in question 'on a bed side in an unseemly posture' and that later the same night Janet said to Richard, 'God forgive you for what you have done to me this night'. (His next try on was that 'he had a design that night & at that time to have committed uncleanness with her, but was happily prevented in accomplishing his design'.) An employer also got involved in the South Leith case (December 1738) of Betty Couts and George Rutherford. Rutherford's master was shocked that Rutherford had denied carnal dealing with her, advising the session that 'that Woman that he is blamed with did come frequently to my shop to him, & he & she went off to Leith together, And when I asked him what he was doing with her, he told me she was his sister'. Another employer in South Leith (March 1736), Mrs Bowman, intervened to prevent the sexual act. Mrs Bowman overheard George Knows and the servant, Martha Lees, 'whispering together a while, & then heard them shutting the Room door on themselves',

> whereupon she went softly, & looking through a slitt in the partition wall, saw her sitting upon a seat, & him standing before her, And suspecting they had a bad Design, she forced open the door & beat her with the Tongs, & taking up the Tankard, threw the ale in his face, & bad him be gone.

Walls were sometimes thin enough to overhear sexual activity. In the case of Marjory Thoms and James Ross in Dundee (February 1793), discussed in connection with attempted abortion in Chapter 4, a neighbour declared that she saw Ross go into Marjory's room 'times without number', and 'there being but a thin partition betwixt her Room & Marjory Thoms', she 'heard her feet upon the Bedside when James Ross was putting her into it & she heard them cohabiting together'. More unpleasant was the case of Susanna Mcpherson and her master, David Bannerman, in Glasgow Barony (January 1777). A woman who lived below their flat, 'with only an unplastered floor betwixt them', heard Susanna Mcpherson crying out 'for shame for shame, vile man, vile man', and Susanna told her the next day that her master was 'struggling with her to be in the bed in which she was lying'. (Another witness had her suspicions raised 'by observing that his servant men did not sleep in the house but in the stable'.)

James Barrie told Dundee session (August 1777) that 'tho he were presently summoned before the next Tribunal he could declare before God that he never had ought to do' with Anne Simpson. However, a witness, Agnes Chalmers, had visited

Barrie's brother and sister one evening and found them in bed together, 'upon which she the declarant went to the Bed & took hold of Anne Simpson & calling her a bad Name desired her to come out of the Bed & she answered she would not for she had torn her Clothes'. In response to this testimony Barrie claimed that he had felt unwell that night and gone to bed, and that Anne came into the bed and would not go away when he told her to, 'to which Agnes Chalmers answered that it could not be so for they were in such a posture as that Anne Simpson could not get away, she being below him'.

Andrew Neil in Edinburgh St Cuthbert's (January 1712) denied fornication with Jane Reid, 'an Idiot'. Janet Cook declared that her son, a deaf boy, came for her and took her to the stable, 'and when she entered she saw Archibald Neil with his breeches down above the poor fool Janet Reid, and her cloaths were up, and it was a considerable space ere he could come off her to put up his breeches: Upon which the declarant said to him, What! are you committing whoredome with a fool.' The trouble was that the only real witness to the act was a nine-year-old boy who was, moreover, deaf, and a mentally defective woman, so the case had to be referred to the presbytery committee for difficult cases.

In some denial cases nothing suspicious had been seen before a child's birth, but the man's behaviour afterwards did not conform to his denial of paternity. In Edinburgh St Cuthbert's (May 1751) a witness declared that Thomas Hay, a married man, who had denied guilt with Margaret Niddery, 'came to his house, and in his Sight gave Margaret a Crown, That he took the Child in his arms & kissed it, and said that maybe there was part of it his' – and that he would help to bring it up. In Glasgow Govan (January 1723) three women declared that David Symm, who denied guilt with Mary Craig, said to the midwife after the birth, 'you are wearied by being up all night fostering my Babie'. And in South Leith James Taylor, who denied guilt with Isabell Bowman in March 1730, was heard responding to her query, 'Is not this child, which is on my knee, yours & mine' by saying, 'Indeed, it is, it is my child'. The presbytery found it proven by witnesses that he acknowledged the child to be his, though it was another few months (November) before he admitted this to the session.

The above might seem to imply that women virtually always named the true father of their child. Sessions rightly did not make such an assumption. Grizel Kyle in Edinburgh St Cuthbert's (January–May 1706) named John Donaldson, a soldier in Flanders, as father of her child, but it was rumoured that the true father was George Andrews, a married man who was also away. George's sister declared that Grizel said to her that 'she never had peace in her conscience since she denied the father of her child'. Confronted with this by the session, Grizel, 'falling a weeping', confessed that she was guilty of adultery with George Andrews.

In the above case there was enough evidence to establish the true father, but often there was no evidence at all. In Aberdeen in August 1746 Margaret Branden first named Walter Leith and then retracted this, saying that 'It was very ill done and that she was sorry she had accused an innocent man'. She said that the real father was Charles Leith, who went away with the rebels, but the session, finding that Margaret 'was exceedingly at a loss in giving Answers to the Session's Queries', doubted this story as well. Also in Aberdeen (May 1763) Isobel Robb first named George Founteroy, then Forbes Gardener, and then Thomas Strachan, a soldier who had gone to North America but denied guilt before he left. In North Leith (December 1759), after first denying being pregnant at all, Isobel Watt named Alexander Moodie as father. When he denied this she said that 'she had accused him out of Spite and Envy, hearing that he or his wife were the first who had told that she was with child'. She then named William Taylor who, she said, had been 'impressed into his Majesties Service', but the session continued dealing with her, 'doubting much if she had yet given up the true father'. (Moodie 'took Instruments in the Clerk's hand that said Isobel Watt had Judicially freed him of being the father of her Child'.)

In one instance the mis-naming appears to have been a genuine case of mistaken identity. When Mary Milne in Aberdeen (September 1747) was confronted with Adam Duff, merchant, whom she had named, she said that 'it was a gross mistake in her to have accus'd him being altogether innocent'. 'The guilt was committed in the silence of the night', she told the session, and 'not knowing the person committing the guilt with her, she asked and was answered that it was Adam Duff'. She had since learned that it was actually James Silver, a married man, under-porter of the college. It is also quite possible that Margaret Forrester, who told Dundee session in march 1774 that her party was 'one of Serjant Sutherland's Recruits', really did not know any more.

But some women told out and out lies. Jean Gamack (a relapse) in Old Aberdeen named the Laird of Troup younger, sheriff depute of Aberdeen, as her child's father in November 1716. The moderator exhorted her 'not to wrong any gentleman... but to be faithfull in the Light of God & man with respect to her confession', but she insisted that it was him. He denied 'any such thing or any scandalous carriage any manner of way with such a woman'. In March she said that 'she did not know the man who begot her with child, save only that he had a blew jockie coat on him, with a silver tressen about his Hat'. Asked why she had accused the Laird of Troup she said that 'it was ill Council that she had gott... & being further pressed by the Moderator who gave her that Ill Council, declared that it was her own evil heart'. In September she retracted her second story as well and said it was James Gilmoir, a married soldier. He was away with his regiment, but a year later he was in town and appeared before the session, denying everything. Witnesses could prove nothing, and eventually the session, finding that she 'had so grossly prevaricat in giveing two or three different Men to be the father of her Last Child & that she still Remained Ignorant Insensible & Unreformed', referred her to the presbytery.

In Dundee in June 1779 Janet Menzie first denied being pregnant and then, when the midwife found her to be with child, said that John Kennadie was the father. He denied this, and in September she declared that she had wrongly accused him and that John Shaw, a married man, was the true father; he too denied the charge, and

> The Session considering that whereas Janet Menzie had formerly given her Child to John Kennadie an unmarried man & endeavoured to prove a Correspondence betwixt him & her by Witnesses but failing therein had retracted her Word & now having given John Shaw a married Man for the father of her Child & proposed to prove a Correspondence betwixt him & her by the same Witnesses which she adduced to prove it with John Kennadie were of opinion that... her word could not be relied on.

Some of those women did eventually tell the truth. Janet Edward in Dundee (September 1754) named Robert Souter, sailor, who had been pressed into the navy and sailed in the spring, leaving money for her with John Murray. The session

7: Lying to the Session

suspected that Murray was actually the father. When she gave birth soon afterwards she named John Murray's half brother, Charles Angus, but a week later she said that Souter was the true father. The session had learned that the ship Souter was on sailed at the end of September, and she was therefore told that 'it was Impossible that Robert Souter could be the Father of her Child he being near three hundred miles [away] when the child was begotten'. She was referred to the presbytery, and more pressure was brought to bear on her, until July 1756 when, 'with abundance of Tears in her Eyes', she confessed the Murray was the father, saying that 'she was a gross abominable Lyer and was heartily sorry for her offence against God'. Murray of course denied the charge.

Much safer than naming someone whose movements could be traced, or who could eventually appear before the session and deny the charge, was to invent a fictitious father, or name a man who had recently died. Jean Henderson came to Dundee session when she was nine months pregnant (June 1779), naming John Wood, 'deceast', as father. As she 'had never informed the Session of her being with child while he was alive' she was told that she would have to produce witnesses who heard him admit this, or the confession could not be regarded as 'genuine'.

Margaret Robertson told Edinburgh Old Kirk session (July 1707) that the name of her child's father was David Johnston, but she 'did not Inquire whose servant he was att the time nor what service he was going to nor how to get an accompt of him'. She did, however, supply the session with the name of his uncle in the parish where she said she had known him previously. The session wrote to the minister there, who replied that there was no one by that name living in the parish who could possibly be the uncle in question. By this time Margaret had disappeared. Isobell Winram in South Leith (August 1756) said that her party's name was David Smith, and that he had been pressed aboard a man o' war, but that she did not know the name of the ship. She added that they had been seen together in Mrs Lyons' house, where the child was begotten; but Mrs Lyons subsequently declared that Isobell was already with child when she came to her house. Margaret Thomson in the same parish (September 1713) did name the ship that her alleged partner, John Black, was supposedly on, but a year later the session clerk managed to track down a member of the crew of that ship, who said there was no one by that name on board recently or listed in the ship's book in the past. Isobel Forbes, a 'trilapse' in fornication, told Old Aberdeen session (March 1745) that her party, John Grant, was the servant of a Mr Bailie living near North Berwick. The session wrote to the minister there, who advised that there was no Mr Bailie or John Grant residing in the parish.

Misinformation could be supplied by the woman's family, as in St Cuthbert's, January 1764. Mrs Abernethy the midwife, called to Isobell Elder in labour, found it difficult to question her, because her father, Thomas Elder, was sending messages and suggestions to Isobell that she should name one or another untraceable highlander who had lodged nearby. Thomas Elder had also tried to prevent any questions being asked during labour. The theory that a woman was bound to be truthful at such a time sustains a knock from Isobell, who named two men, including one of the highlanders, in her labour. She later claimed, when she named a third, that she had not known what she was saying when in agony. The session, not surprisingly, considered that none of the three was the real man.

An alternative to creating a fictitious father was to claim an attack by an unknown man. Agnes Coul in Glasgow Barony claimed in August 1764 that she had been attacked by an unknown man but in October named James McKimmen, saying that he told her to 'Say that it was begot by some body upon the road, And not be bleat with the Session.' It was not surprising that sessions rarely believed such stories.

Janet Downie told Edinburgh St Cuthbert's session (July 1776) that 'a man who was a mason & drunk' got her with child in her brother-in-law's house, that she 'made no resistance nor called upon the neighbours for Protection' and had not seen the man before or since. The session judged this story 'Utterly Improbable'. Some women embroidered their stories with more detail. In October 1716 Christian Clerk, a St Cuthbert's parishioner, said she could not name the father of her child because one night in April when she was going to get pigeons out of the dove-cot

> there came a man to her when it was a little dark, cloathed with a Red-Coat, & a Rough Cap on his head and spoke strange Language to her, which she understood not, having a drawn sword in his hand, and violently threw her down, and stop'd her mouth when she offered to cry out, and committed Uncleanness with her.

In her case and in the cases above the woman had not related the circumstances to anyone at the time they happened. Even in a genuine case this would not perhaps be so surprising since – as seen in Chapter 4 – a woman would be considered guilty even if she had resisted, whereas if she did not become pregnant no one need ever know.

Although in the overwhelming majority of cases the story of an unknown rapist was fiction, obviously such a thing could happen. In January 1703 Margaret Brown told Old Aberdeen session that a man on horseback whom she had never seen before or since 'lighting from his horse forc'd her to committ uncleanness with him in the Links'. When asked if she knew his name she said she did not but that 'when she came to Tarbathill she was informed he had been there & made his vaunt how he had Ravished a woman in the Links'. This boast proved his undoing, for he was traced and proved to be Mr William Dalgarno, apprentice apothecary. He was cited before the session and Margaret recognised him as the man.[6]

In one case where the man in question was not traced the woman's story was nevertheless believed. Eupham Johnstoun told Edinburgh Old Greyfriars session (July 1713) that she was delivering a letter to a carrier in the West Bow for her master when she was assaulted by two men who 'appeared to be officers, having silver lace upon their coats, and swords about them'. Elders spoke with her master who said that on the day in question he told her off for staying out so long and she replied that 'she hade been fasht with two men in the west bow'. Others who knew her declared that 'they never observed any lightness in her behaviour, and that she was opprest with grief and sorrow upon the account that she should be with child not knowing the father thereof'. The midwife testified that at the time of her pains Eupham had declared she had been forced by two men, and Eupham declared that 'she could with the greatest of freedome take ane oath thereupon if desired'. The session referred the case to the presbytery (February 1714) which did 'not find ground to proceed against her for any thing that yet appears'.

The procedure which was to be followed in such cases was precisely laid out:

> If a woman who had brought furth a child does Declare she knows not the father alleadging she was forced as in the fields by a person unknown, or any the like reason in these Caices great prudence is to be used the former behaviour of the

7: Lying to the Session

woman exactly searcht into, and she seriouslie dealt with to be Ingenuous, and if she has been of entire fame she may be putt to it to Declare the truth, as if she were upon oath, but not without the advice of the presbyterie and no formall oath should be taken, and if the woman Confess she was not forced, but does not know the man, whether married or unmarried, the same Censure is to be inflicted upon her as in the Caice of Adultery.[7]

In all of the above cases, and many others, where a woman claimed an unknown or untraceable man as father she was ordered to make her public appearances as an adulteress in sackcloth. However, sessions did use their own discretion. In May 1749 Margaret Elmslie was referred by Aberdeen session to the presbytery because she could produce no evidence that a soldier by the name of Bevenhouls was the true father of her child but refused to appear in sackcloth. But a week later the session decided that they had 'ground to believe that she is ingenuous in her Confession' and allowed her to appear in the ordinary way.[8]

Women who did not reveal the name of their child's father faced the humiliation of appearing before the congregation innumerable times, in sackcloth, while their partners got off scot free. So why did they do it? One answer to that question is clear from the case of Agnes Bannerman in Old Aberdeen. In November 1731 she had claimed that the father of her child was a dragoon. In March 1739 she was dangerously ill and wanted to confess the truth, that Alexander Anderson was the real father. She declared that

he lay with her in his own Barn, yea sometimes left his wife in bed & would come to her, that his wife discovered their criminal correspondence & put her away at Candlemas from her Service, That she would have confessed the Truth before now but he threatned to murder her if she gave him for the Father of the child & that she was really afraid of his threats as an accident of that kind happened in Aberdeen a little before she went home to his service, but as she had now the near views of Death her Conscience would no longer allow her to conceall the Truth be the Consequence what it will.

Agnes was not the only woman who feared for her safety. In Dundee Janet Crab was apprehended after giving birth alone in her room and exposing the child, though she continued to deny all this until threatened with imprisonment. She then admitted everything, '& being asked the reason she continued so obstinate in refusing to confess the truth Answered that John Low threatned to Kill her and the Child if she should give him up as the father of the child'. Grizel Morison delated herself to Edinburgh St Cuthbert's (October 1720) as guilty with Charles Straton. When she told him she was with child to him he

bad her gett a broken Sailer whom she never saw before, to father her child upon, [and furthermore] he threatned to kill her, if she would not father her child upon another, and she promising accordinglie for fear of her life… but she thought that the oath she made to him… was unlawfull, and it was no sin for her to break it.

However, more usual than threats were bribes, emphasising the disparity in the positions of the men and women involved. Isabell Mar said to Old Aberdeen session (September 1742) that after she told James Skeen, son to the Laird of Lethentie, that

Sin in the City

she was with child 'he declared that he would take care of her, only she behoved not to expose him'. He gave her twelve shillings sterling, telling her it was six weeks provision at two shillings a week, '& That he would from time to time give her money, providing she took Care of his Character'. He, of course, denied all this, and she later said that 'he had begg'd her to give up his servant John Brown as the Father of her Child, and he would give her money, & further that the said Brown had come to her, desired her not to give her bastard to His Master but to him & promised to take with it.' The session considered all this and presumed 'there behoved to be some foundation in Truth'.

Elizabeth Brown in Glasgow Govan (January 1749) said that Allan Scott 'offered her some money to go out of the place untill she had brought forth the child'. A witness declared that at Scott's behest he 'Desired her Rather than affront Allan Scott she should give the child to another father'. Another witness declared they heard Scott telling her that his own father would withhold money from him and refuse to allow him to support her and the child, whereas if she accused someone else 'she might be sure that Mr Scott would not allow her to want and that this would be much better for her'. (The 'Mr' of course meant gentry status.) Agnes Durrie in Aberdeen (February 1760) was sent for to the house of an advocate who 'offered her a Guinea or Two not to Father her Child on Andrew Duncan Alledging that it was better for her to have a full Basket than to stay in Town and attend the session.' And Margaret Reid told Glasgow Barony session (May 1771) that James McNair younger sent for her and said that 'he would give her Money and a Letter to go to Edinburgh and that she should want for nothing if she would give her child to another man'. (Witnesses heard him offer her money, and the session judged him guilty.)

Many more examples could be given. In Aberdeen (August 1779) when Janet Beidie, who had gone to her home parish, appeared before the session she said that Thomas Black 'had given her half a guinea to give the child to another, and also that when she acquainted him that she was going to leave the Town he said she ought to have gone away much sooner, and gave her five shillings sterling to bear her expences'. In the same parish Jean Begg (June 1779) said that two months earlier an advocate offered her 'both Gold and Silver which he held in his hand if she would sign a paper which he then produced, and told her the Contents of it were to declare that Mr Bannerman [also an advocate] was not the father of her Child and that she should give it to some sailor or soldier or gentlemans servant or any absent person, but she refused to sign the said paper.'

It cannot have been easy for women to resist such pressure. Margaret Campbel had twins and named James Ranny, cooper, as father. He denied this to Edinburgh St Cuthbert's session in November 1725, in response to which Margaret said that the previous Thursday night James was in Helen Scobie's cellar and sent for her. At that time 'he told her he would own the Children & appoint a factor for them while abroad, providing she would keep the matter Secret, and this very day he sent a Cadie for her to come up to the same Cellar none being present with him & her save the said Helen Scobie, & then & there he wrote & sign'd a Line to her for Fifty shillings sterling & gave her the same upon condition that she would not compear before the Session this day to which she acquiesced'. But when she got back to her own lodgings her landlord 'advised her not to absent from the session in case he denied his guilt with her & to evite that she compeared'. Ranny insisted that the 'Line which she pretended she got from his 'tis forged', but the session 'were

7: Lying to the Session

convinced that he was the father of the Twins'. Helen Scobie, who had overheard their conversation, appeared at the session's next meeting. She said that James 'promised her a new plaid, if she would advise Margaret to father the Children upon some seafaring man', which she refused to do. He finally confessed, claiming that Margaret and Helen Scobie 'were the occasion of his prevaricating in regard they both told him that if he would give Margaret a piece of money, she would gett another father to the Twins.'

Of course, threats and bribes were not mutually exclusive. Sir James Nicholson, named by Elizabeth Crae in Edinburgh New Kirk (August–November 1713) apparently looked after their child but did not compear before the session. She said he told her that 'he was very willing to give her a Guinea and Mount her with good Cloaths upon Condition she would goe out of the Kingdome, so that he might not be any more fasht about that Child'. Later he had 'urged her mightily to sign a paper Declareing He was not the father of the child all which she refused to grant and finding he could not prevaill with her to condescend to any of his proposalls he swore he would cause putt her in the correction house, and there force her to live on bread and water And said that whenever he gott his opportunity he would cutt the child in collops so that he should not be fasht with him or her'.[9]

The above have all been cases where a woman ignored a threat, or refused a bribe, or took the bribe and then came to the session anyway, and named a man. But what of all those women who never came up with the truth and who made numerous appearances in sackcloth? Christian Reid in Edinburgh St Cuthbert's (April 1756) could perhaps be taken as representative of them all. She had named an unknown man, and after her child was born the session learned that 'she was some way supported above what could be expected from any shift she can make under the burden of Child which she is nursing'. But enquiries proved fruitless, and she then absconded, presumably well looked after by her protector.

What about cases where a man denied guilt, and there was insufficient proof to judge him guilty, though too much suspicion to allow him to swear an oath of purgation? The usual procedure was to suspend the whole case, merely narrating the story to the congregation. One of the Aberdeen ministers strongly objected to this, in May 1744. Jane Johnston had named William Craig, merchant in Glasgow, as her child's father. He had denied this and claimed that she was commonly reported to be a 'Strumpet'. The session discovered that she was no such thing, but the presbytery advised that 'there appears to them to be no ground to fix the scandal' on Craig, and so a narrative of the case should be laid before the congregation. The moderator was unwilling to do this, because it meant that if a woman was unable to prove her accusation the process regarding both her and the man would be suspended, 'even tho' the man delated by any such woman be of equal bad Character with William Craig of whose ill Report the Session are not ignorant; And altho' the Session shall not be able to fix the Character of a Common Prostitute upon the woman accusing as they have not upon the strictest enquiry been able to fix on Jean Johnston.' However, the presbytery insisted and the following month a narrative of the case was read out to the congregation.

Many denial cases are far too drawn out and complex to be related in this chapter but too fascinating to be left out of it, so Appendices 3–8 provide some case histories.

The conclusion to be drawn from the contents of this chapter is that the

Sin in the City

mechanism of social control drawn up in the sixteenth century – and which worked reasonably well in rural Scotland through much of the eighteenth century – was inadequate when it came to a rapidly urbanising society. The clergy and elders did their best, but the status of many male urban dwellers, and the sophistication of all ranks in the cities, made is possible for them to run rings round kirk sessions and presbyteries.

Notes

Edinburgh, Canongate and Leith kirk session registers are in the Scottish Record Office; the only exception is Edinburgh New Kirk which for the year 1706 is in Edinburgh University Library and for several other years in Edinburgh City Archive. Aberdeen St Nicholas registers are in Aberdeen City Archive; Old Machar registers are in the parish church, with access via Aberdeen University – microfilms of both sessions' records are in the Scottish Record Office. Glasgow Barony and Govan session registers are in Glasgow City Archive, and have not been microfilmed. Dundee registers are in Dundee City Archive, with microfilms in Edinburgh. We have not given references for each citation but always state the month and year, making it possible for anyone to find a particular case.

1. In February the kirk treasurer had declared that Walker came to him about a fortnight before the woman was cited, '& dealt with him to conceall the womans being with child, & offered to give him a Bond of four pounds sterling, if he would do it'. In October, after his confession, Walker 'desired the Session would delay his publick appearance, till his Apprenticeship was near out'. The session agreed to the delay, but claimed it was so 'that he may be dealt with in order to his being brought to a deep sense of his sin to prepare for his publick appearance'.
2. Christina Larner, *Enemies of God* (London, 1981), p. 103.
3. In April 1723 Gray produced another extract, from the city guard books, that the previous January she had been committed to the city guard 'as a Common whore, and found in a Badie house'. He continued to deny guilt with her but acknowledged that 'it was not prudence in him to be in the said Margarets Company'. The session decided that she was 'not ane object of Church Discipline'; Gray was rebuked sessionally.
4. The case of Margaret Taylor and William Hay, merchant, could have been used as a precautionary tale of the perils of the big city for innocents from the country. When Margaret arrived in Edinburgh Hay approached her, and she recognised him as having called at her mistress's house in his travels. After 'asking after some of the people in Caithness whom she knew and professing the greatest kindness and friendship for her and offering to serve her in getting her into a good place in Town, he pressed her and insisted with her to go into a house with him to get a Refreshment upon which they went in together and he called for a bottle of wine to drink, & she drank a share of two bottles of wine which made her very sick and much out of order, upon which the Landlady put her to bed which was in the room and left him and her together and upon this she cried for help from the house but the Landlady called to her that she needed not to be afraid for he would do her no harm and so after much opposition that she made he at last got his advance of her and debauched her and so she has fallen with Child'. She was subsequently able to take some elders to the house where it happened.
5. Mary Batees in January 1715 told the session that intercourse occurred in June and that 'Mistris McLeud sent for her... and when the said Mary came to her, told her that there was a friend in her house that desyred to see her, and that the said Mistris Mcleud put her into the room where the said William Paterson was, and then she retired'. Mary added that

Paterson gave her two shillings sterling immediately afterwards. Mrs Mcleud was cited before the session for 'tripanding' Mary; she denied this, but Mary said that 'she did send a young boy who was barefooted for her'. Mrs Mcleud 'could not deny but that there was such a boy staid in her house', and the boy declared that he had gone for Mary.

6 A complication in this case was that while giving birth Margaret named another man as father, George Umphra. Umphra denied guilt but in January 1704, 'being interrogat if he was willing to purge himself by oath... answered that he could not deny but that he uncovered the nakedness of the said Margaret & that being a particular clause of the oath was not willing to perjure himself'. He too was therefore ordered to appear publicly.

7 Extracted from Old Greyfriars session register 24 August 1713.

8 Most sessions demanded evidence of an absent man being the true father of a child, either by witnesses' testimony or by a letter from the man; if this was not forthcoming then the woman was either left under the scandal (i.e. not allowed to appear publicly) or made to appear in sackcloth. However, Aberdeen session consistently allowed such women to make their appearances if there was no evidence of their guilt with any other man. For example, with regard to Mary Crawfurd (October 1739), 'The session considering that her Confession is very probably genuine and true' allowed her to make her appearances, and in fact the man she named returned to the parish and confessed three years later. Other examples include Isobel Hosie (July 1722), Anne Elphinston (July 1752), and Jean Milne (December 1762).

9 Sir James eventually appeared and denied guilt. Soon after that Elizabeth Crae retracted her previous confession of his being father of her child, but later at the same meeting said that Sir James 'dealt with her to deny what she had formerly confest and for which he promised her money'. The case dragged on for years, but once she had disappeared (amply compensated no doubt) it became harder to establish the truth. Five years later (September 1718) he petitioned the presbytery, protesting his innocence. The presbytery committee for difficult cases 'were of opinion there is not sufficient ground to proceed to any Censure against him unless some other evidences of his guilt appear'.

Appendix 3

Case History 1: Aberdeen

15 January 1705:
Helen Aiken confesses fornication, declaring that the father was 'a Gentleman in drink Rideing upon a horse with a footman of whom she Interrogate his name who said it was Robert Forbes but that she knows no more of him never haveing seen him before nor since'. The Session, 'perceiving clearlie that she did grosslie prevaricate', appoints her to be kept in prison to stop her absconding.

22 January:
She says that the father was actually Lewis Maitland who has gone to the East Indies. After giving details of where and when it happened she is asked if she has any evidence, 'such as if he had ever spoken to her formerlie anent committing uncleanness with her or if he had given her or promised her anything upon her yielding to his desire'. She says she has no evidence and that it only happened once. The session think that if he really was the father she would have spoken sooner as he left the country on 22 September. More pressure is put on her to tell the truth, and she then says she was guilty with him not once but three times. The session has 'great ground to suspect that as yet she is not Ingenuous'.

1 February:
She declares 'most solemnlie' that it was Alexander Forbes of Cregie, 'Merchant in this Burgh and late Bailie, a married man', saying that he sent a man to her while she was in prison who 'counselled her to give her child to Lewis Maitland and not to Cregie'. She adds that she told Maitland's mother when she came to her in prison that she was guilty with Cregie and had also told the town clerk when she was first imprisoned, and that the previous day, Alexr Leslie procurator fiscall to the Sheriff Court came to her in prison... and bade her retract what she had said anent Cregie otherwise it would goe verie ill with her and that Robert Mowat weaver heard him as she thinks and bade her stand to the truth and not to retract.'

5 February:
Cregie denies and Helen retracts her accusation, saying 'she was Imposed upon by Mistress Angus and Mrs Brown to Nominate the said Alexr Forbes of Cregie and withall added that the said two persons perswaded her... that she would not get out of prison till Lewis Maitland came home if she did not clear the said Lewis & give to the said Alexr Forbes and that if she would give it to him she would presentlie win out of prison as also added that at that tyme she would have given it to any bodie to get out of prison'. When asked about the confessions she had made to Maitland's

mother and the town clerk she admits making them, 'but withall now adds that it was an untruth that which she did say and that she thinks the Devill tempted her'.

12 February:
The session examines witnesses. Elizabeth Maitland declares that she went to the house of Maitland's mother, and Cregie came in and spoke to Maitland's sister, Anna, 'and that the said Anna Intreated her Mother in the Deponent's presence that Helen Aiken might to be advised to give her Child unto her Brother Lewis Maitland... perswadeing her thereto by saying it would ruin a mans Familie and break his wifes heart if the child were not given to the said Lewis Maitland upon which the Deponent declareth that she went unto the prison window where the said Helen was and said to her that she was now allowed to give the child she was with unto Lewis Maitland and that the said Helen answered let them doe what they pleased for she had confessed to no body but Clerk Thomson... and therefor desired the Deponenet that she should goe to the Clerk and desire him to be silent' and she had done so. But later, 'being Exceedinglie grieved for being any wayes accessory to the Nomination of the forsaid Lewis Maitland that she went to the prison... and Intreated her to tell the truth for she would have nothing to doe with it'. Anna Maitland and her mother refuse to appear before the session; they, and Cregie, are referred to the presbytery.

19 February:
Cregie appeared before the presbytery and continued to deny. Maitland's mother and sister did not appear, but Anna now appears and depones at length. She insists that Cregie never proposed naming her brother Lewis and never confessed guilt with Helen to her but that 'haveing heard that the forsaid child was given both to Lewis Maitland and to Cregie she thought her Brother being a free man it was less hazard to give it to him than to Cregie a married man'.

28 May:
Helen 'hath been publicklie disgraced and Banished the Town'.

29 October:
Cregie is to be laid under the sentence of lesser excommunication but gives in a paper offering to purge himself by oath.

4 March 1706:
The moderator reports that Cregie confessed his guilt before the presbytery.

Appendix 4

Case History 2: Edinburgh St Cuthbert's

1 January 1708:
The session had received a letter from Dunbar stating that Jane Wilson accused John Clerk, 'stockin weaver', a married man, as father of her child. She now appears, with her father as cautioner, and says that 'he enticed her to the wickedness one day when she mett accidentally with him att the fountain-well in Edinr she then serving one Mrs Johnstone a change-keeper on the Shore of Leith, and when they mett together at the fountain well aforesaid, she craved him for a chapine of wyne, which he took on in her Mistress's house in Leith, because they would not change him a Guinea, it being a time when the Guineas were passing at a lower rate than formerlie, but he bad her goe with him, and he would pay the chapine of wine, whereupon they went together up the street, and he took her into a Change house in harkerstoun's wynd, where they drank together, and ate some Collops, for which he payd two shillings Scots, and confessed she was guilty of Adultery with him in that house in a closs room, the door being shutt and the Land Lady of the house was angry at the declarant when she desired that the door might stand open, and Declares the said Land-lady came and satt down beside Mr Clerk in the bed-side of the room, and said to him O Mr Clerk, you are a great stranger! and that Clerk took the said woman about the neck and kissed her fourty times, and the woman seemed to entertain his carriage kindly'. She says that that was the only time she was guilty with him and that she told him when she knew she was with child to him: 'Then said he God damn him eternallie if he would take with it, but he entreated her to say that Robert Clerk once his apprentice was the father thereof, who was now off the Country, and perhaps would never return again, and if she were called to it, he bad her swear it, but she answered that she would not swear it, but would say it, but Mr Clerk replied, that swearing was nothing, for many ane oath he had sworn in his time. And at another time being big with child she came to the said Mr Clerk, he bad her expose the child: but she answered, she would not take upon her to be guilty of Murder, and he again bad her fix the guilt upon Robert Clerk, who was abroad.' Her father tells the session that he had gone to Clerk regarding the baptism of the child and 'Declares that Mr Clerk bad him tell his Daughter to come to town to gett the child baptized with an Episcopal Minster for five pence or fourteen pence or the like'.

22 January:
Clerk claims she was guilty with another man, John Laing. She denies this.

Appendix 4

29 January:
After witnesses' depositions the session, clearly believing Clerk to be guilty, refers the case to the presbytery.

Subsequently: The presbytery believes him guilty. He continues denying and is laid under the sentence of lesser excommunication.

Appendix 5

Case History 3: Aberdeen

21 October 1723:
Christian Tellie, whose child was born in September, confesses that she is a trilapse in fornication and names William MckGee, who she says is 'a Caithness man of no fixed residence'. The session thinks she is 'prevaricating'.

11 November:
She now names Alexander Kempt, senior mason, and says she was induced to name MckGee by him, 'but now, for the ease of her conscience, she was content to tell the truth'. She says that when she told Kempt she was with child to him he first told her to go to her aunt in London, and then to name MckGee as father, 'and after that she resolved to go south and bring forth her child, & when she came to Stonehaven, she heard that the said Alexander Kempt was working at Fetteresso, & sent a boy for him, and he came… and said he had little money to spare, however he gave her half a crown and two shillings sterling and six pence, & told her, when she sent him word of her delivery, he would come & see her, Though it were fourty miles distance from this place, & would give her money from time to time, & ever since she was put in prison, he hath sent her money by her mother'. She says he was also the father of her last child and that 'thereafter did lye carnally with her severall times', and that 'when she came to be in courtship with one George Gilchrist sometime servant to Baillie Gellie, & got a ring from him worth a guinea, he the said Alexander Kempt, upon her acquainting him with so much, diverted & diswaded her from going on with the said George Gilchrist in that matter, telling her that it was not a fit bargain for her, & bad her delay a while, until his wife, who was an aged frail woman, should die, and that then he would marry her, & that would be a better bargain for her & withall added that the said Alexander Kempt told her, that if she gave him up as the father of any of her children he had begotten with her in uncleanness with her, that he would confidently deny it before Magistrates and Ministers, & finally added, that upon her mother's signifying her displeasure in his coming so frequently about the house, when she was with the second child, & putting him to the door, he thrust the door up again & did strike both her & her mother… as the people thereabout can declare when called'.

19 November:
She says that when she was in prison her mother told Kempt that she would not be able to conceal his name any longer, and that he had offered to pay two pence out of every sixpence he earned if she would continue to conceal it. She gives in a list of witnesses who saw them together. Kempt appears and denies everything.

Appendix 5

23 December:
They both appear. He is told that the session is ready to hear anything he has to say and to witnesses on his behalf, but he refuses to offer anything, whereupon the session prepare to hear her witnesses and Kempt refuses to stay. Numerous witnesses depone. One, a weaver of 37, says that on King George's coronation day in 1714 they were in Christian's mother's house, and Christian and Kempt were there when Kempt's wife came and from the door and, 'in the deponent's hearing, cryed out, come out you adulterous dog & you adulterous whore, I have found you out'. Another witness, an excise officer, declares that one night about two years ago he had attempted to enter Christian's mother's house and when he finally got in he found that 'they had barriceaded the door with daills, trees and a form, and having gone and looked about him, saw Alexander Kempt lying among the peats'. He had then pursued Kempt, 'calling to him by his name Alexander Kempt, and saying Alexander this is wrong, this will make all good that is said of you, & that he the deponent pursued him so hotly that he the said Alexander Kempt losed his hat & wig'. Many others declare seeing them together.

30 December:
Kempt has appealed from the session to the presbytery on the following grounds: '1o/ Because I received not a full extract of the confession & the articles of the delation given in by Christian Tellie against me 2do/ Because what Note of a libell or delation I got with the names of witnesses was not given me in due time, having only received the same three lawfull dayes before the meeting of the session, Whereas I should have received them at least ten dayes before, 3to/ Because when I compeared befor the Kirk Session, and offered by grounds of exculpation from the scandal raised against me, with a list of witnesses for proving the same... they utterly refused to admitt the same... 4to/ Because they went to the examination of witnesses, notwithstanding by my appeall I secluded myself from the privilege of being present... By which it is evident, how greatly I am prejudged by the said forward procedure of the Kirk Session'.

6 January 1724:
The session's answers to the above begin by stating that the presbytery will easily see that 'his appeall is most preposterous'. Regarding the third point, 'it cannot but be thought very strange, and it is hoped will be noticed by the Reverend Presbyterie, that the said Alexander Kempt should presume so far as to misrepresent the conduct of the session in the state of matters of fact'. As for the fourth, it was he who refused to stay and hear the witnesses, although 'he was desired again and again to consider what he was doing'. After reading a full extract of the session's procedure, and witnesses' depositions, the presbytery found his appeal 'most preposterous and litigious'.

17 August:
He is placed under the sentence of lesser excommunication. Christian Tellie is to be proceeded with according to her confession.

19 years later (13 June 1743):
Kempt confesses guilt and the sentence is lifted.

Appendix 6

Case History 4: South Leith

21 June 1733:
Elizabeth Young says the father of her child was John Crawford, Collector's Clerk in Bo'ness. 'Said she has received three Letters from the said John Crawford unsubscribed & a Twenty shillings note with one of them. And that four days after she delivered of the child, she with the child were after Ten of the clock at night transported to Edr in a chair, attended by two men whom she knew not, but understands one of them is called Leven, And when she came to Edr she was lodged some nights in Duncan Lindsay's house in Roxburghs Closs there, Said the child is now nursing in the house of Archbald Campbell Chairman at the Butt Closs opposit to the Tron Edr.'

19 July:
The session have had a letter from the minister at Bo'ness stating that he had received the extract of Elizabeth's confession, 'And that John Crawford Clerk of the Customs there, having been examined, denyed what she charged him with, being encouraged thereto by a Letter under the said Elisabeths hand, dated at Leith 22 June last… in which Letter she retracts her confession… & frees him of any accusation for her Misfortune of having been with child, And alledges the ill usage she gott from this session, together with her low condition made her in such confusion as to agree to any thing they pleased right or wrong.' The session has also received a letter from Crawford denying guilt with her and stating that the letters she mentioned had been transcribed by him 'for & at the desire of Mr Lobhan. Complaining also upon this session for threatning her with prison, if she did not name him & no other for the person guilty'. The session has to admit that 'it is true that the said Elisabeth Young did… at first name one John Crawford a wright lad in Edr as the father of the child, who, she said, was gone to the West country, & whom she had not seen for six months bypast, & could neither tell where he was, nor to whom he belonged, nor with whom he wrought when at Edr. And this, with the way & manner of her being clandestinely removed with her child from hence to Edr under cloud of night so soon after her Delivery, & being there concealed for some time, made this session suspect her Ingenuity [ingenuousness] in the matter, and therefore threaten to deliver her to the Magistrates to be secured, untill she should give a true account of the father of her child, And then she made the confession as it was transmitted to Borroustouness, which seeming more probable, the session in their Minute took no notice of her having first named a man whom she could give no account of'. Elizabeth appears '& owned her writing the Letter to Mr Crawford of the 22 June, & with Impudence adhere thereto, but Denyed that part of it to be true wherein she writes that she was

threatned with prison if she did not say that the child was to Mr Crawford, of Borroustouness, & owned that the session neither bad her name him, or threatned her if she did not name him.' The midwife declares that when she was giving birth Elizabeth 'with uplifted hands Declared then that John Crawford Collectors Nephew in Borroustouness, & none other, was the father of her child, otherwise she wished she might never be separated from her child, nor see the face of God in Mercy. And when the Declarant saw the said Young some time after she had been before the session, she asked her, how she could give a wrong father to the session, & Young answered, But they caused me tell the truth ere all was done'. George Lobhan, custom house officer at Bo'ness desires access to the session and admits transporting Elisabeth in a chair from Leith to Edinburgh and taking the child to a nurse, but says that the letters were written 'for John Crawford the Wright' and says 'he knows John Crawford the Wright, & that he is now in the North Country, & has Letters under his hand owning the child'.

21 February 1734:
John Crawford, Collector's Clerk in Bo'ness, confesses guilt.

Appendix 7

Case History 5: Edinburgh St Cuthbert's

20 June 1734:
Barbara Robertson appears of her own accord, saying she had brought forth a child and the father was William Pearson, linen cloth dyer. She says intercourse happened twice, the first time in the field of Pilrig late at night 'and at that time he was so very rude to her that he dragg'd her like a Dog when he committed the Lewdness'. After her delivery on 12 May William sent his friend, Neil Campbel, and the kirk treasurer's man, who 'took away the child from her, and gave it to the Nursing, and after her recovery Neil Campbell gave her Two Shillings Sterling, and bad her goe over the water to abscond, and also payd the Midwife in whose house she delivered'.

27 June:
Pearson denies. The moderator reports that he had lately received 'a paper sign'd by the two initial letters of her name, which when read, did sett forth that what she had last day confessed before the session as to her adultery with William Pearson was contrary to her Conscience, and it was out of spleen she so stain'd him because he withheld her wages from her, and seeing she is a dieing woman she cannot burden her soul with such a horrid sin, as to blame the Innocent, Therfore now Declares, that the Child she has brought forth is to James Smith Late servant to John Forester Cordiner on Caltoun & to no other, and the postscript of the letter bears, that if this will not satisfie, she will send the session word where she is, and Declare the above-written herself, all which the session suspect to be Trick and Cheat and that Wm Pearson has Industriously Imposed upon her to keep him from Censure; The Moderator sharplie rebuked him for practising with her in such a manner, which greatly aggravates his wickedness; and withall told him that this Session would not so easily pass it, but would prosecute him to the utmost'.

4 July:
Pearson denies again and says he knew nothing of her letter, 'neither does he know where Barbara Resides, and Suposes that it is out of Malice that she Loads him with the Guilt, because he would not give her money for she said that if he would give her a shilling, she would not fash him.' The kirk treasurer's servant says that on his master's orders he took the child to be nursed 'because it was starving, and Barbara brought the child to him'; he knew nothing of William Pearson. The midwife says that while giving birth Barbara named a young, unmarried man, James Smith, and denies receiving payment from anyone.

Appendix 7

7 July:
Neil Campbel refuses to testify.

11 July:
Pearson protests that he is not obliged to appear before session or presbytery as his accuser had acquitted him and named James Smith. The session represent to the presbytery a number of reasons why he must be made to answer, including the fact that 'Barbara herself did freely own both to the Elder and Deacon of the district that both Wm Pearson and Neil Campbel concurred together in desiring her to father the child upon the same James Smith', and John Forrester, the alleged master of James Smith, said he never had such a man in his service.

1 August:
Barbara appears 'and Declared that what was written in the letter… was nothing but a trick put upon by the midwife Mrs Courtess who brought her to bed who dictated both the letter to the Moderator & another to Wm Pearson and a man whose name she knows not wrote them both, and Mrs Courtess led her hand at the Signing of them because she cannot write herself, and before Subscribing of the Letter directed to William Pearson he said to her if she would signe it, she would never want all her Life as Long as he was here… and Wm Pearson with the midwife perswaded her to father the child upon James Smith & now declares that she knows no such man, for the saids persons had imposed upon her, and further declares that Neil Campbel gave the midwife Mrs Courtess for bringing her to bed Twenty five shillings sterling'.

3 October:
Pearson has given in a petition to the presbytery alleging that Barbara's accusation proceeded from malice and that in view of her prevarications it should be invalidated; Barbara has given in a petition to the presbytery giving presumptions of his guilt. The presbytery remits the case back to the session to investigate further. Pearson's witnesses are cited to this meeting but none appear.

14 November:
The session advise the presbytery that Barbara has answered all of the session's citations while Pearson has ignored them.

26 December:
The presbytery finds that the presumptions do 'not amount to a proof of his guilt with her'. A narrative of the process is to be read before the congregation and the case is then to lie over until providence give further light. She is to be censured as a adulteress according to her confession.

Appendix 8

Case History 6: Glasgow Govan

7 December 1777:
Janet Speirs names Matthew Liddle as father of her child and alleges that he promised to marry her.

14 December:
A witness declares he heard Janet say to her parents that 'if her father would give him his Watch he would marry her directly.' Her father declares that Matthew 'had agreed to take breakfast with him upon the Wednesday following in order to finish the affair, that accordingly he came and took breakfast and promised to meet him in Glasgow which he did not perform'. Matthew's mother insists that he denied that the child was his. 'It being alledged that she shook hands with the Woman and wished her Gods blessing declares she does not remember whither she did it or not for she was in a Confusion.'

22 February 1778:
A witness – Margaret Sweetman – alleges that Liddle acknowledged to her that he was the child's father. 'The Moderator desired her to hold up her hand and make Oath that he might put the proper Questions to her she absolutely refused to make Oath.' Liddle's mother 'likewise absolutely refused to make Oath.'

1 March:
The first witness says 'The womans words were that Matthew had told her that if her father would buy him a Watch at three Pounds and put her well off the House he would marry directly'. The next morning 'the Deponent... believed that from what had passed the night before and from what he now saw he believed that he not only acknowledged the guilt but that he designed to marry her instantly.' Janet alleges that Liddle's sister said to her that 'it was a heartless doing to her but that her brother James Liddle whatever way it would go would see to her'. Janet also alleges that Liddle's sister and mother sent for her 'and her Mother said where will we get a house for you and that Lad upon which the Deponent [Liddle's sister] said that they would get the House below'.

3 August:
Liddle's mother and Margaret Sweetman appear. 'The Session reasoned with them and finding that they seemed to have no inclination to declare the truth' decide to delay the matter.

30 August:
'The witnesses seemed… to be as backward to declare the truth as ever. The Session were very apprehensive that both these women being so closely connected with Liddle would rather injure themselves than declare the truth thought it inexpedient to examine them upon oath. The session are informed that the Village of Partick are in general impressed with a sense of his guilt and leave it to the Presbytery to finish this matter in the way that to them shall seem most expedient.'

5 December 1779:
The moderator asks Liddle, who has been before the presbytery, 'what he had to say and if he was going to exhoner his Conscience and confess his guilt with Janet Speirs who was also present accusing him as before, he refused all guilt with her And produced a Paper the Prayer of which was that the session would instantly administer him the Oath of Purgation. The Moderator called upon him to consider the importance of his request especially as there was a Proof of many presumptions of his guilt And advised him to take three weeks to consider the affair seriously and then come again and report to the session.'

21 May 1780:
Liddle appears and 'penitently acknowledged that he had been once guilty of the sin of Fornication with Janet Speirs And that on the same Day that she alledged But had long denied guilt because he apprehended the Child could not be his as it was three Weeks above nine between the commission of the guilt and birth of the Child And declares that he is now sorry for his conduct and that he has given so much trouble to the Presbytery & Session.'

8

The Rise and Rise of Irregular Marriage

The seemingly inexorable rise of irregular marriage was arguably the aspect of urban life that made kirk session control of the populace more difficult than any other.[1] Regular marriage meant the proclamation of banns on three successive Sabbaths and a ceremony by the minister in the parish church. The very public nature of regular marriage would deter bigamy and thus be a safeguard for women in particular.[2] But a marriage did not have to be carried out in this way in order to be legal. Dating back to canon law in the Middle Ages, all that was necessary for a valid marriage was the free consent of both parties. If there were no legal impediments then the mutual statements 'I take you for my wife' and 'I take you for my husband' in the presence of two witnesses was as binding as a church ceremony, as was a promise to marry followed by sexual intercourse, which was taken to imply present consent.[3]

The main constraint against rushing into marriage was the expectation that a couple would be financially independent and able to set up house together. This was a major constraint in rural areas, but in cities servants did sometimes marry, cohabit briefly in lodgings (which established the marriage), and then return to their employment. Girls in towns also married soldiers and sailors who might disappear for years afterwards.

Before the eighteenth century the overwhelming majority of marriages were 'regular' ones. The Church bore down hard on couples who did not conform. An Act of 1661 against those who married 'in a clandestine way' threatened offenders with three months' imprisonment and a sliding scale of fines from 100 merks to 1,000 pounds Scots, according to rank. In 1698 a further Act penalised the witnesses to irregular marriages and the men conducting them.[4] There are a few seventeenth-century cases recorded in the register of the Scottish Privy Council, based on attempts to get hold of heiresses,[5] and a few in the records of Trinity College parish, Edinburgh, of those of lesser rank. Of nine cases recorded in Old and New Aberdeen, seven were by Roman Catholic priests, and so was one of the two recorded in Edinburgh Canongate parish. In other words, at that time the main motive for irregular marriage was basic religious divergence from the established Church.

The situation changed radically after the Revolution of 1688–9. As discussed in Chapter 1, the establishment of Presbyterianism forced more than two-thirds of the incumbents of Scottish parishes out of their posts. Hundreds of unemployed ministers were seeking other sources of income, and many of them gravitated to Edinburgh. For anyone who did not wish to get married in the conventional way, alternatives now presented themselves.

Sessions were annoyed not only at marriages being conducted without banns being

8: The Rise and Rise of Irregular Marriage

called, but also at the tendencies of the celebrators to put false information on the certificate. Antedating it was usually done to avoid a charge of antenuptial fornication, but other falsehoods appear to have been sheer devilment. Samuel Mowat appeared before South Leith session in December 1701 for this offence. On the certificate for John Young and Janet Ingles there were 'three direct lies': he had stated that he married them at Musselburgh, but the couple declared they had been married at Leith; he stated that they were married on the first of July while they declared they were married on the sixth of September; and finally he stated that William Tait, cooper, was witness to the marriage, although Tait declared before the session that he was in Holland at the time of the marriage. In the 1690s the names of Samuel Mowat and James Kirk predominated; from 1701–20 the name of John Barclay appeared most often on marriage certificates, and in the 1720s it was Gilbert Ramsay. The fact that the same names appeared again and again on irregular marriage certificates was in fact very useful to kirk sessions, because the handwriting could be recognised and forgery ruled out. When in 1754 a St Cuthbert's couple produced marriage lines signed 'Patrick Douglas', 'the session considering that they had never seen Marriage Lines of his before refused them as documents'. (Douglas's name appeared regularly on certificates after that.)

From the 1730s onwards celebrators of irregular marriages were no longer Episcopal ministers. In that decade David Strang (sometimes spelled 'Strange'), a Presbyterian minister dismissed from a northern parish for misconduct, held almost a monopoly on irregular marriages. Strang was particularly prone to cock a snook at authority by making various statements on his certificates without verifying any of them with the couples being married. For instance, according to the certificate produced by Janet Bruise and Thomas Fogo to North Leith session in July 1734, they 'solemnly declared that they were free persons had the consent of friends and were not within the degrees forbidden in Gods word'. The couple admitted they had signed the certificate but denied 'that any such questions were asked'. Strang became such a major irritant to the Church that action had to be taken. The presbytery laid him under the sentence of lesser excommunication in 1735 and greater excommunication in 1737. North Leith session took additional action. In June 1737 couples were still going to Strang to get married, in spite of his lying under the sentence of greater excommunication, 'to the open Contempt of the Laws of the nation both Civil and Ecclesiastick', so the session decided 'to put a stop to such Irregularities by Censuring such Delinquents in a more public manner than by a sessional Rebuke' and ordered that henceforth all couples married by Strang would have to appear publicly.[6] That did not, however stop them from resorting to him.

In 1738 the civil authorities intervened, and David Strang was imprisoned in the Tolbooth. (He then had the gall to petition the presbytery 'that some method may be thought upon for his Subsistence'. The presbytery, noting that he had broken every promise he had ever made, instead set up a committee to urge full legal action against him.)[7] Even this did not stop him, for couples came to him in prison to get married. In December 1742 year it was reported in the presbytery that notwithstanding the fact that David Strang 'is under sentence of Banishment for his Marrying persons contrary to the Law, yet he continues in his Irregular practice.' By this date David Strang's name rarely appears on marriage certificates, but North Leith session noted in November 1742 that Elisabeth Gray and William Blyth's certificate were married by David Strang although the certificate was signed 'David

Sin in the City

Williamson Minister the name now assum'd by the said Mr Strang'. In November 1743 one minister moved that the presbytery 'order some charitable supply to Mr David Strang, Prisoner in the tolbooth at Edinburgh', but when the ministers of South Leith produced a marriage certificate recently signed by Strang, the presbytery rejected the motion.[8]

David Strang died in the Tolbooth in 1744,[9] and no single celebrator ever held a monopoly again, but a colourful character was popular in the 1740s. In May 1737 David Paterson was still a probationer (i.e. not yet a qualified minister) at the Tron Kirk when he was accused before St Cuthbert's session of being the father of Janet Dods' illegitimate child. He denied the charge, although he had promised the Kirk Treasurer of Edinburgh – in writing – that he would accept financial responsibility for the child. The session continued to press him to confess while he continued to deny. In October of the same year Paterson was one night found to be concealing another woman in his house. Suspicious neighbours had attempted to get in, had called the baillie and officers, and asked 'who was with him? he answered what is that to you, and refused to open the door, tho' they frequently called for access, & would not open it till it was violently broke open by an hammer & a chezil by violence'. He denied being guilty of fornication with the woman to St Cuthbert's session, and when 'the moderator asked him the cause & ground of bringing Isabel to his room? answered it was to give her his Linnings [linens] to mend, & when asked if he said to the magistrate that he could not want [do without] a woman? answered it might be he said so for he knew it to be the case of some men & it might be his case also perhaps'. Continuing to deny guilt, he was asked 'if he attempted to committ Uncleanness with her? he said he had not time'. He was referred to the presbytery, 'but Mr Paterson was pleased very obstinately to answer that he would not answer the Presbytery, and does not regard the Summonds.'

David Paterson was placed under the sentence of lesser excommunication in January 1738, which might have deterred a lesser man, but instead of a career in the ministry he set himself up as a celebrator of irregular marriages. In August 1742 the constable of the Abbey of Holyroodhouse told Canongate session that Paterson had taken a room there 'where he continued the practice to marry persons irregularly, and sometimes three or four Coupel in a Day.' The presbytery gave him his first admonition of the sentence of greater excommunication in June 1741, subsequently gave him a second and third admonition as well as ordering prayers for him, but finally, in January 1743, 'found no Evidence of his Repentance or Resolution to amend his ways' and therefore passed the sentence against him. As with David Strang, this had no effect on his trade as a celebrator of irregular marriages, though North Leith session again insisted that persons married by this 'excommunicate person' appear publicly before the congregation. In the 1750s he was in prison but still marrying couples from there.[10] In 1758 he was mixed up in a scheme to claim that a common prostitute had been married by him to a recently deceased gentleman and therefore had a right to the gentleman's estate. It was then stated that 'the said David Paterson had been for many years not only a Reproach to the Ministeriall orders but had been and still continues to be a perfect Nuisance in the Town and City of Edinr and suburbs thereof where he still lurked notwithstanding of a Sentence of Banishment pronounced against him by the high Court of Justiciarie'.[11]

In Glasgow the commonest celebrator's name on marriage certificates was John Smith. But one woman producing a certificate with that signature to Barony session in September 1747 said that 'to the best of her knowledge it was Mr How that Married them, for she was since in his shop, and when she lookt at him thought he was the same person that married them'. In December of the same year another couple 'both declared That although the Lines be signed John Smith That the man who married them was James Lorimer Baxter in the Bridge-street Glasgow.' Was there a real John Smith? We do not know. Perhaps he was a business consortium.

The whole business got even murkier when some Edinburgh session clerks started earning cash on the side by providing out of town couples with documents allowing them to marry in the city. In August 1742 James Gilchrist and Helen Birrel, parishioners of South Leith, obtained a document stating that they had been legally proclaimed, on the strength of which they were married by one of the ministers in the city. In January 1743 a committee appointed by the presbytery to consider this problem, suggested that an elder or deacon be required to identify all persons before they could be married. But such abuses continued. In September 1747 the minister of Lamington parish complained to Canongate session that their clerk had given a certificate of proclamation of marriage to a couple 'as residing in the parish of Canongate' who had in fact continually resided in Lamington, and they too had been married by one of the Edinburgh ministers on the basis of that. The couple were 'both of very bad character', which explains why they went to Edinburgh and why the Lamington minister was particularly outraged. The clerk insisted that he had been imposed upon by someone's telling him that the man was 'of a sober character coming & going to the place'. In November the session decreed that the clerk was prohibited from proclaiming anyone until the kirk treasurer was satisfied that one or both were resident in the parish.

The most persistent offender in this regard was Mr Dunning, session clerk of St Cuthbert's. A South Leith couple got a residency certificate from him in November 1754, and though the man said he had 'imposed' on the clerk 'by the pretence of possession of a room in that parish', Mr Dunning was involved in other shady deals as well.[12] Dundee session complained in November 1762 that two of that town's parishioners had obtained residency certificates from the session clerk of St Cuthbert's; the Dundee clerk considered their marriage 'illegal & surreptitious', though the session eventually sustained it.

Twenty five years later (Jan 1787) another Dundee couple were married in Edinburgh after obtaining a residency certificate from Trinity College session clerk, although they had told him frankly that they were Dundee residents. In response to Dundee's complaint Mr Lundie, the Edinburgh minister who had married the couple sympathised with the complaint, explaining that 'the Ministers of Edinburgh could do nothing in that matter – they having no power over the Session Clerk he being chosen by the Magistrates & supported by them'.[13] This is another illustration of the erosion of kirk sessions' control by the end of the eighteenth century, and it also shows again that couples who chose to marry clandestinely could easily do so.

But why did couples choose to get married irregularly? In England many apparently did so to avoid expensive and elaborate marriage festivities.[14] This motive does not appear to have operated in Scotland. To prevent riotous drinking and dancing 'penny' weddings, the usual form of party after a marriage, were forbidden, and the 'consignation money' paid by couples at proclamation was returned only if there was no unseemly and boisterous party after the wedding (and a child was not born less than nine months later). Also, couples had the option of marrying 'privately' instead of before the congregation if they paid a little bit extra.

Sometimes there were obvious practical reasons for secrecy and speed. Sailors might expect to be called to sea at short notice, and soldiers might fear being prevented from marrying by their officers. In April 1712 two men who had married irregularly appeared before Edinburgh St Cuthbert's session, saying that 'they were unwilling to take such an irregular course, but each of the men being soldiers in fflanders they gott orders to make ready for sailing in the moneth of March and had they taken the ordinary way of publication of banns, they thought they would not had [sic] time.' Sessions certainly wanted to prevent such abuses as experienced by Janet Meekie in North Leith (Dec 1738). She had married John Blanket, 'a stranger and weaver to Trade'. After the clandestine marriage she had taken him to her house 'where she beded with him all that night and on the Sabbath morning they went up again to the Cannongate where he robb'd her of her plaid and [she] never saw him since'.

A Scottish marriage did not require the consent of parents to be valid. However, many parents felt that their consent *ought* to be a legal requirement; in October 1758 one Edinburgh couple advertised in the local paper, the *Evening Courant,* that their children, if they married against their parents' wishes, as one had already done, would be disinherited. Financial pressure was also exerted on John Story, who admitted to Glasgow Govan session in December 1763 that he had promised to marry Agnes Robertson before getting her with child, but that 'his Parents were very averse to the Marriage and threatened that if he married Agnes Robertson they would turn him out of their house and give him nothing.' To what extent this was an excuse for his own reluctance to marry we cannot know. However, when a couple who had been married by David Strang in March 1733 came before Dundee session and were asked if they had their parents' consent 'answered they hade not for hade they hade that they would not have troubled Mr Strang', which suggests that this might have been a fairly common motive.

But the commonest motive of all appears to have been something we can only term 'fashion'. In certain decades there were quite simply far too many irregular marriages for any other explanation to be valid. In South Leith during the 1730s and 1740s in some years there were more irregular marriages than regular ones.[15] North Leith session noted in May 1730 that 'all of the marriages which have happened in this parish since the current year commenced are clandestine & that none have been duely proclaimed in the church', and again in September 1731 that 'a very few of a Long time have been married in that Decent, regular, & publick manner, as the Laws of the Nation both Church & State do allow'.

The period when it was in fashion varied in different parts of Scotland, as can be seen from Appendix 9. (There were never any local celebrators in Aberdeen, so a journey to Edinburgh was necessary for any couples there who wished to get married irregularly.) Dundee's peak was clearly in the 1770s. South Leith's was the 1750s, after which there were certainly more regular than irregular marriages. The session recorded all marriages, regular and irregular, in the 1770s and 80s: from 1774–9 23 per cent of marriages were irregular, while from 1780–5 only 8 per cent were irregular. But even in the same part of the country differences abounded. It is clear from the Glasgow Barony figure for the 1780s that the fashion was far from over there, and in fact in November 1805 Glasgow presbytery sent a questionnaire to all the parishes within its bounds, asking if irregular marriages were frequent, increasing

8: The Rise and Rise of Irregular Marriage

in number, and had given rise to 'illegal and criminal connections'. Govan session answered 'no' to all three questions, while Barony answered 'yes' to all three and noted that in 1784 there had been 12 irregular marriages in the parish, in 1794 there were 23, and in 1803 there were 46 (which implies over 400 irregular marriages in the decade).

'Illegal and criminal connections' meant bigamy, and indeed a significant proportion of irregular marriages were bigamous.[16] A plausible newcomer to the neighbourhood might con a woman into marrying him, and of course celebrators of irregular marriages did not demand proof of single status. Women who had been deserted many years earlier would have to provide evidence of their husband's death before being allowed to be proclaimed for marriage, which was a powerful incentive to marry irregularly in hopes that the local kirk session would not remember the earlier marriage. The Church was to some extent trying to protect women from being exploited but at the same time created hardship.

Divorce was available in Scotland for either husband or wife on the basis of adultery or desertion. But desertion had to be 'wilful', and the deserted spouse had first to prove both marriage and desertion and sue for 'adherence' before the consistory court, as well as petition the presbytery, so there were not many suits on that score. In our rural study we did not find divorce mentioned as an option, but in Edinburgh we did encounter divorced couples. (A man or woman divorced for adultery was not allowed to marry the co-respondent, and such couples continuing to cohabit attracted the attention of ecclesiastical courts.) Although an uncontested divorce case for adultery could be completed within three months, and some individuals were allowed the benefit of the poors' roll, overall it appears that the costs of legal action put divorce out of reach of the majority.[17]

Urban sessions were certainly aware of the possibility of divorce. In September 1706 Margaret Russell, spouse to James Ker, tailor in Edinburgh Trinity College, was with child to a soldier. Ker 'declared that he and the said Margaret Russell his spouse hath not cohabited together these three years past & desired to be divorced from her But the Moderator told him the session cannot divorce him, for it belongs to the Commisar'.[18] The most extraordinary judgment was that of Edinburgh presbytery in January 1718. Janet Thomson and James Crawfurd appeared before Edinburgh St Cuthbert's session for irregular marriage although his first wife, Janet Dunlop, was still alive. The presbytery advised that after reading of the process,

> having considered that Janet Dunlop his first wife was guilty of Adultery, and absconded more than six years agoe, and being informed that the said James has not cohabited with her ever since the said Crime was committed, and made evident both before the Presbytery and Session; are of opinion that there is a reall tho' not a Legal divorce, from one another, there being nothing wanted to have the Legal one perfited save money on James his part to prosecute the same before the Judge Competent he being in mean circumstances. Therfore the Revd presbytery think fitt that the session should overlook the affair betwixt James Crawfurd and Janet Thomson.

Such a common sense approach was unique. Far more usual was the reaction of North Leith to a similar situation in September 1735. Agnes Munro and George Tilloch were irregularly married while his first wife was still alive. He produced a testificate 'of her being convict of the crime of Adultery before the session And

Attestation by William Paton late Baillie of an Intimation made by his order by Tuck of Touns drum Discharging the Inhabitants to Harbour or Entertain her But the session finding no step for a divorce in Law' referred the case to the presbytery. Tilloch insisted 'he was not in any capacity to prosecute a Divorce in Law against his first wife', but the presbytery forbade him to cohabit with Agnes. Similarly, John Bartie petitioned Dundee session in October 1779 'shewing that whereas his wife had left him & been guilty of Adultery he was designed to marry another & therefore wanted the Advice of the session upon that Head the session having considered the same were of Opinion that they could give no advice in the matter unless that he should take out a Divorce as he could not marry another till that was done.'

Because divorce for adultery did exist, it was arguably one step to the belief that the adultery was equivalent to the divorce. James Wynd in Dundee, who had married Jean White, acknowledged to the session in December 1776 that 'he had a Wife in Aberdeen but thought she had divorced herself by going away with another Man'. Similarly, James Rowand in Glasgow Barony was married to Margaret Richie whose first husband, James Marshel, was still alive. In June 1785 Rowand said that as Marshel 'had gone away with another woman from Margaret Richie about two months after their marriage he imagined that James Marshel's adultery dissolved the marriage with Margaret Richie & that she was at liberty to marry the declarant'. The session prohibited him to live with her 'till she obtain a regular divorce from James Marshel & can be regularly married.'

Sessions often learned of bigamous marriages through the first wife appearing before them. In July 1752 Elizabeth Benstead came all the way from London to South Leith to complain of her husband, James Adams, marble cutter, who had deserted her twelve years earlier and was now living with another woman. Although she produced a marriage certificate Adams insisted that 'he never knew or saw the said Elizabeth Benstead, till within these few weeks that she came to Scotland, That she is an Imposter and the Certificate produced by her a forgery contrived and conducted by the Malice of his Enemys who envy his Success & want to cutt him out of his Trade in this place. That he never married any woman but Janet Bruce his present lawful Wife.' The session wrote to someone known to them in London who inspected the register of marriages and found the first marriage registered in accordance with the certificate produced.

A more convoluted case was that of Mary Partridge in Glasgow Barony (March 1765) who came from Ireland, swearing that William Smith married her about five years ago and sent for her at harvest last. She said that she had lived with him since then 'as his acknowledged wife, but that lately she had been made to understand that he has another wife at Falkirk upon whom he had been regularly married before he sent for her the Complainer from Ireland, And that he now acknowledges the Falkirk wife, But refuses his Marriage with her the Complainer'. Mary was able to produce plenty of proof of her marriage, and the session, 'perceiving this affair of Smiths to be plain Bigamy', did not consider itself a competent judge to proceed further, 'But in regard the said Mary Partridge is manifestly wronged & injured by said William Smith her husband his Marriage with Elisabeth Gillespie at Falkirk The session appointed their Clerk to give to said Mary an Extract of this whole affair as it lies before them... That she may use the same as she shall think expedient in procuring a Redress of the wrong done her as law will'.

Some women were conned into marrying a man who had a living spouse, but some were well aware of her existence. Women also married bigamously, though they did so less frequently than men. Sometimes a woman simply did not know whether her husband was alive or not, but a sizeable proportion of both partners who entered on a bigamous marriage did know. Means of communication were limited, and there was ground for hope that the truth would not emerge. George Chalmers, irregularly married to Elizabeth Stephen, was asked by North Leith session in July 1757, 'how he could pretend to Marry a Woman who had another Husband alive?'. He replied that the man was reported to be dead, 'and upon the bare report of his death they adventured to Marry, nor as yet was there any thing known to them, but that he was dead'. The session clerk then produced a letter from a contact in London stating that her first husband was alive and in good health, 'and wants to be commended to his said wife' – 'after hearing said Letter they were somewhat confounded, & said what could they do now as they were so long Married, and the woman with child'. They were, of course, forbidden to cohabit. Similarly, Helen Bain told the same session in August 1765 that she had heard that Alexander Kirkwood, her previous husband, had died four months before she married Alexander Wylie. 'The session were by no means satisfyed with this answer as severals of them had reason to believe, that said Alexander Kirkwood was still alive att Glasgow. On hearing of which said Helen Bain stood speechless.' In both those cases one cannot be sure if the couple were confounded at the session discovering the truth, or whether they really had believed their stories. Either way, they had not taken sufficient trouble to establish a former spouse's death and were therefore forbidden to cohabit.

In Glasgow Barony (Nov 1744), Margaret Graham was asked if she had formerly been married to Thomas Scot, a soldier; she acknowledged giving the session marriage lines in 1741, having claimed at that time to be married to him, but now insisted that 'Scot wrote the said Lines himself and that there was no marriage between them; But that she had cohabited some time with him in Uncleanness'. Five weeks ago she married James Gemmill, weaver, who acknowledged being married to her. The case was remitted to the presbytery who found that Thomas Scot 'never judicially acknowledged' his marriage to Margaret. The session cited witnesses in an attempt to establish whether the couple had been married or not. A local barber declared that Scot and Margaret had told him they were married, and showed him their marriage lines, and also went to bed together, and cohabited for three or four weeks, 'at which time he was taken up as a Deserter and carried off the Country'. There was therefore no doubt that the second marriage was bigamous, and as the couple continued to cohabit, in February the presbytery went so far as to pronounce the sentence of greater excommunication upon them. A few weeks later Gemmill expressed his repentance and abandoned Margaret (though rather than face public censure he left the parish).

Bigamy cases could be lengthy and complicated, and space prohibits a further discussion of them here, but Appendices 10–12 provide case histories for three of them.

One thing clearly illustrated by the case of Margaret Graham, Thomas Scot, and James Gemmill, is that whereas there could be little doubt about whether a marriage which had been publicly proclaimed, and performed in a church, was valid, irregular marriages could be far from clear cut. Although the consistory court was the final recourse for proving the validity of any marriage, urban kirk sessions had constantly

Sin in the City

to try and establish whether a couple could legally cohabit. The need to define what precisely constituted a true marriage provides some of the most fascinating material to emerge from these records.

As noted at the beginning of this chapter, according to civil law, if sexual intercourse followed a promise of marriage then a marriage had been made, as legal and binding as any made in a parish kirk. The Church, however, did not follow this line. Many women alleged a promise of marriage by the father of their child, and sometimes the man admitted making the promise and subsequently changing his mind, but sessions treated this as any other case of fornication, and the child was considered illegitimate.

An exception to this occurred in Dundee in October 1777. The beadle reported that Elizabeth Miln had been sent out of town by her father 'in order to prevent her marrying the Man to whom she is with Child'. Elizabeth and the father of her child, William Thorn, appeared before the session and produced lines which they had written and signed in January of that year in which Thorn swore to God that he would 'never marry another Woman as long as Elizabeth Milln lives, but her', and Elizabeth swore likewise, 'To which lines both parties adhered & declared them to be their own hand Writing which they voluntarily wrote & signed': 'The Session considering that whereas said parties had thus mutually & voluntarily bound themselves to one another by the above mutual Obligation to which they still adhere & the Woman being with child in consequence thereof they could not look upon them in any other Light than married persons – they were accordingly declared married persons by the Moderator'.

In April 1780 Margaret Sime's marriage proclamations in Dundee were stopped because the session was informed that she had a husband alive. She denied this, acknowledging only that 'she went away with a Man to be married & staid Six Months as his Wife'. But the session had heard that 'she came home with Child & gave out that said Child was to her Husband', and decided that 'her having staid so long with a Man as his Wife & brought forth a Child to him as such would constitute a Marriage & therefore unless she could prove that the Man was dead she could not be married to another'.

However, unlike commissary courts, kirk sessions did not refer to precedents but came to their decisions in a remarkably ad hoc manner. For example, in a similar case in Canongate in February 1747 a different conclusion was reached. William Shaw, invalid soldier, who had recorded his name for proclamation of marriage with Janet Hog, was reported to have another wife alive. He admitted cohabiting with Margaret Baillie for four or five years and that she bore a child to him but denied being married to her. Witnesses were cited. A soldier in the same regiment declared that though Shaw and Baillie had indeed cohabited for some years, 'the Declarant alwise looked upon her to be his Whore and not his Wife, but owns that the said Baillie during that time, bore Shaw's Name as his Wife to screen her from being drummed out of the Regiment as a Whore, and that the said Baillie owned to the Declarant that she was never married to Shaw'. Another fellow soldier concurred and declared that 'he knew the said Baillie go off afterwards with a soldier in the old Buffs, and that when she left him she married another soldier in Sackviels Regiment… and that he the Declarant signed as Witness to their Marriage, having never looked upon Baillie to be married to Shaw or else he would have been far from

8: The Rise and Rise of Irregular Marriage

doing it.' The session treated Shaw as a fornicator and allowed his marriage proclamations to go ahead.[19]

A similar situation occurred in North Leith. In December 1760 Isabel Boon, who had left the parish some time ago with a soldier, 'as his wife', returned without the man and was asked if she could produce any documentation of her marriage to him. She 'declared that she did cohabit with a soldier in this place for the space of nine nights, that they were Married as soldiers for the most part do, by taking one anothers word, but that he was long gone from her, and as she hears has taken two or three wives since.' She was ordered to appear publicly three times for fornication and then to remain under the scandal, as she was known 'to have been all along a lewd woman'. It is questionable whether her soldier really did think his succession of women to be 'wives'; from the Canongate case it appears more likely that he considered them to be his whores, and that when he came to take a 'wife' then some kind of ceremony would take place.[20]

Not that a ceremony was any guarantee that a valid marriage had taken place. In October 1753 South Leith, faced with a request for marriage proclamations from a man who was rumoured to have irregularly married another woman, asked that woman what had occurred. She said that in November 1751 she had happened to be in the house of Andrew Bowman in Canongate, where William Smith was at the time, and that Bowman brought a man to the house 'who spoke some Words which she did not understand, but took them for a Joke'. She declared that Smith had at one time courted her, but she had never consented to marry him, so when he 'told her that she was married to him by the said man, & proposed to bed with her, she refused both, being at that time under promise of Marriage with William Hunter her present Husband with whom after regular Proclamations she was married in a few Weeks thereafter'.

In Glasgow Barony (April 1745) it was reported that James Clydesdale and Elizabeth Davie had been declared married persons by an acquaintance of theirs, James Meiklejohn, in the presence of witnesses. Elizabeth denied being married and said that on the night in question Meiklejohn had declared that he would marry them, and a member of the company had forcibly put her hand into Clydsdale's. Meiklejohn had said he did not know not 'what words to pronounce. But at the last said Ye are married persons'. He then 'threw the covering of the Bed over them while they were still sitting together in Token of their being Bedded.' The couple in whose house this happened confirmed her version of events and declared that the whole thing 'was purely done in jest, and flowed from the greatest part of the company being the worse of drink.' Meiklejohn expressed remorse and was 'sharply rebuked for his Drunkenness and what happened in the consequence of it, and told if ever he was found in such a practice again he would be prosecute with the outmost rigour of law.' This seems a bit extreme, but in a case in the same parish in January 1765 a man tried to stop a woman's marriage to someone else on the basis of a similar kind of 'ceremony' three years earlier. Once again the session judged that no marriage had taken place.

In our other Glasgow parish, Govan, there was a report in March 1763 that John McKenzie and Janet McFarlane had been married by William Davidson, weaver. Janet agreed that this had happened while John denied that any marriage had taken place. David Anderson was a witness:

> Depones that they sat for some time and that the Woman and Man took [each] other by the hand That Davidson in a Laughing manner said that they were married persons. That afterwards he the Deponent went to Door and when he returned the Woman was gone to Bed in the same room where they had been Drinking and that he was present and saw John McKenzie go to Bed to the said Janet McFarlane... Depones he saw William Davidson make up some sort of Lines which he called Marriage Lines.

Davidson 'being asked whether in a jocular manner he said they were Married persons Depones he does not remember whether he said so or not... But said to them that if they went to Bed before witnesses that that would make them married Persons'. Basically, if both parties had intended to be married then Davidson was quite right; the difficulty arose when one party genuinely believed themselves to be married and the other did not.

In South Leith (April 1719) Helen Spence produced a certificate of her marriage to William Beveredge, signed by a well-known celebrator, Gilbert Ramsay, but Beveredge insisted that 'if he was Married, he knew nothing of it for he was Mortally Drunk, & that the man who Married them was as Drunk as he was, & said that he never cohabited with her as his wife And that he did not bed with her that night'. Helen admitted the latter fact, 'but averred that he did cohabit with her since as her husband.' Witnesses subsequently declared seeing the marriage, but Beveredge still insisted that 'he was beastly drunk & ensnared into it', and that he did not cohabit with her but 'was only in her house as a Lodger'. The case was referred to the presbytery for advice.

In Glasgow Barony (Sept 1769) Hendrie McIndoe denied being married to Elizabeth Nicolson, who had borne his child. As she was able to produce witnesses who heard him call her his wife, and as he had obviously bedded with her, the session was clear that the couple were 'to be considered as Husband and Wife'. McIndoe appealed against this to the presbytery, but the presbytery upheld the session's decision. Similarly, Alexander Wallis denied being married to Janet Stewart (North Leith, Aug 1769), claiming that his signature on the marriage certificate was a forgery. There were witnesses to the marriage, and the couple had cohabited, so the Session was 'of opinion that there is sufficient evidence produced of their having been irregularly married, but being an ecclesiastical court they cannot compel the Man to cohabit with the Woman, and therefore leave the matter to be decided by the proper Judges'.[21] The following year Wallis was irregularly married to another woman, a marriage which the session refused to sustain as valid.

Sessions certainly did not uphold every claim of marriage. Elizabeth Gabriel told South Leith session (June 1726) that she was married to William Purse but that he had taken the marriage certificate with him when he left the parish. However, he had written a letter to the kirk treasurer in which he averred that 'the Report & talk of his being Married with her was the occasion of his leaving the place & going for London & from thence to New England, owns that he has Lyen with her as his whore since the month of May before but Denies that ever they were married'. Elizabeth was unable to find any witnesses to the marriage, and she was forced to satisfy discipline for fornication. There was a witness to the ceremony between Ann Ritchie and the man who denied being married to her (James Winning) in Glasgow Barony (Nov 1774). The witness had found the celebrator for them and declared that 'after the deponent and the aforesaid man came to James Winning's house they Danced

8: The Rise and Rise of Irregular Marriage

Several Reels and Drunk Several Drams and a considerable Quantity of punch by which means he became considerably headed with Liquor that before they parted he heard the aforesaid man who had been brought into the company make some kind of Speech mentioning the fear of God in it but does not Remember any other word spoken by him.' Neither did he remember the couple joining hands, but he declared that 'it was his Opinion that what passed at that time was a Marriage betwixt the parties... and that he believed it was considered as such by the parties themselves.' However, as no one had seen the couple in bed together, the session concluded that 'there was not sufficient proof of any marriage betwixt them.'

In all of the above cases it was the man who denied being married, which comes as no great surprise, but Margaret Wishart was unusual in various ways. In August 1707 she was referred from South Leith to Edinburgh Old Kirk session. She was 'big with child' and said it was begotten in fornication by Peter Pringle in Edinburgh. She had previously brought forth three children, first to John King in Cupar, Fife, 'about twelve or thirteen years ago', for which she had satisfied discipline, secondly to James Henderson in South Leith, and the third, in Dirleton parish, to John Forrest, 'who is now a souldier abroad'. There were letters from Forrest to her, addressing her as 'his dear and loving wife', 'hoping to see her shortly in Scotland, and if not, promising to send for her', but Margaret claimed that though she had cohabited with him before he went to Flanders she was not married to him. She admitted that 'he called her his wife But she never called him her husband nor never wrote to him Designing him her husband.' Margaret was clearly a law unto herself.

There were many other cases of sessions having to attempt to determine whether couples were married or not, and three more examples are given as Appendices 13–15.

How did sessions learn about irregular marriages? A very few couples came forward voluntarily to register the marriage. More usually elders and deacons would learn that a couple were cohabiting and because – at least until the breakdown of discipline – couples did not openly cohabit without being married, they would be cited for irregularly marrying and asked to produce marriage lines. The time lapse between irregular marriages and citations by a session is a good measure of the grip which that session had on its parishioners (see Tables 8.1–8.3). Looking at either end of the spectrum, the deterioration in the church's control is very evident, particularly in St Cuthbert's. Between 1711 and 1720, 42 per cent of irregularly married couples were cited less than one month after marrying, while only 6 per cent had been married for more than nine months. By the 1740s only 15 per cent were cited within a month and 34 per cent had been married for longer than nine months.

In North Leith control was maintained much longer. Between 1711 and 1720, out of 62 irregular marriages, 60 per cent were cited less than one month later, and only 5 per cent were cited more than nine months later. In the 1740s the proportion caught early was halved, but at 31 per cent was still much higher than St Cuthbert's; 21 per cent were caught after nine months, so there was still a large number cited between one month and nine months after marrying. Even as late as the 1760s, out of 106 marriages, 30 per cent were caught under one month, while 28 per cent were cited more than nine months after marrying. (This information is not given for a large enough number in the following decade.) South Leith between 1711 and 1720 has a much lower percentage caught under one month, though only 8 per cent were over 9

Sin in the City

months pregnant before being cited. The complete switch is by the 1770s when out of 110 marriages, only 8 per cent were cited less than one month after the marriage, and 64 per cent were cited more than nine months (in some cases two or more years) after they were irregularly married.

Table 8.1: Numbers cited at different periods of time after an irregular marriage: Edinburgh St Cuthbert's

	0–1 Months (%)	1–3 Months (%)	4–9 Months (%)	9+ Months (%)	Total sample
1711–20	37 (42)	30 (34)	15 (17)	5 (6)	87
1721–30	34 (41)	19 (23)	20 (24)	9 (11)	82
1731–40	23 (27)	18 (21)	25 (34)	15 (18)	85
1741–50	14 (15)	20 (21)	28 (30)	32 (34)	94

Table 8.2: Numbers cited at different periods of time after an irregular marriage: North Leith

	0–1 Months (%)	1–3 Months (%)	4–9 Months (%)	9+ Months (%)	Total sample
1711–20	38 (60)	14 (22)	8 (13)	3 (5)	63
1721–30	27 (38)	16 (22)	15 (21)	13 (18)	71
1731–40	28 (31)	21 (23)	27 (30)	14 (15)	90
1741–50	31 (31)	20 (20)	29 (29)	21 (21)	101
1751–60	37 (40)	14 (15)	27 (29)	15 (16)	93
1761–70	32 (30)	19 (18)	25 (23)	30 (28)	106

Table 8.3: Numbers cited at different periods of time after an irregular marriage: South Leith

	0–1 Months (%)	1–3 Months (%)	4–9 Months (%)	9+ Months (%)	Total sample
1711–20	33 (30)	26 (23)	43 (39)	9 (8)	111
1721–30	29 (24)	36 (30)	35 (29)	20 (17)	120
1731–40	39 (19)	50 (25)	67 (34)	43 (22)	199
1741–50	61 (23)	62 (24)	74 (28)	65 (25)	262
1751–60	76 (28)	51 (19)	84 (31)	56 (21)	267
1761–70	54 (26)	23 (11)	48 (23)	83 (40)	208
1771–80	9 (8)	12 (11)	19 (17)	70 (64)	110

Early in the eighteenth century one means which sessions used to attempt to control irregular marriages was to refuse to sustain a marriage until the witnesses also appeared before them. As those witnesses would have to pay a fine, there might be

8: The Rise and Rise of Irregular Marriage

some reluctance on their part to obey. One celebrator of irregular marriages, Alexander Irvine, used his son as a witness; as he was only 13 the session did not accept this as valid.[22] A witness to the marriage of Janet Kindy and James Dickson in North Leith (Apr 1719) declared that 'she did not subscrive the Testificate, but a little Lassy did it for her, who was to get two pence Sterling for her pains'. Edinburgh Tron session had great difficulty with two witnesses to the marriage of Catherin Stewart and William Chapman in April 1728. The names of John Blackadder and Andrew Buchanan appeared on the certificate as witnesses, though they had not signed. Both denied being present. This dragged on for some time until May 1729 when the minister who had performed the ceremony appeared before the session at the same time as Blackadder and 'affirmed to his face that he was present'. John, 'being desired to Depone desired some time to think on it'. After that he refused to appear before them again and the case was referred to the presbytery.

Glasgow Barony session continued to lay great stress on witnesses long after Edinburgh sessions had given up. In April 1746 when William Lindsay and Jean Buchanan said they could not bring the witnesses to their marriage because 'they knew none of the Persons that were present at it,' the session refused to sustain the marriage. (The witnesses were eventually tracked down and were produced in November.) In October 1747 Barbara Carr and James Moffat declared that the only surviving witness to their marriage was in 'a dying Condition'. The session took the matter seriously enough to send some elders to call on him; the elders subsequently reported that the dying man 'solemnly declared to them that he was present at the Marriage betwixt the said parties.'

By the late 1750s Glasgow Barony session was no longer interested in witnesses to the marriage ceremony but demanded witnesses who had heard the couple publicly acknowledge themselves married persons; the marriage was considered to date from then, no matter what date a certificate bore. (The session's attitude toward marriage certificates in the 1760s is clear from the reiterated statement that various couples 'produced the ordinary sham lines.') But the session gradually accepted that there was no real need for someone to officiate over a marriage. In May 1764 a couple declared that 'they were married by no administrator But had mutually betwixt themselves two plighted their faith to adhere to each other as husband and wife & had both subscribed the same with their hands... and had consummate the whole by bedding together.' The marriage was accepted as valid, as were two others (in March 1767 and May 1768) who said that no one had married them (though they had witnesses to their bedding).

In the 1770s Glasgow Barony session developed a new procedure for couples who had no real proof of having been married by simply having them sign a declaration of their being married persons. (When one or both of the parties could not write, the moderator read the declaration to them and signed on their behalf.) The session then retained the document and recorded the marriage as of that date. This avoided any possibility of either party later denying the marriage and seems an admirable way of dealing with irregular marriages (though one which could only be carried out by a session still in control of a parish). Yet it also accepted that the only essential thing to a marriage was the consent of both parties.

In the 1790s Dundee adopted its own procedure, which was to intimate irregular marriages to the congregation; if no objection was made then the marriage was sustained. In July 1800:

Sin in the City

> On considering the case of James Butter & Janet Glendie and having read the lines which the parties had acknowledged were written with their own blood, the tenor whereof follows 'March 1st 1800 This declares our Marriage & cited with our blood James Butter Janet Glenday none to witness but God himself' – and being informed that Janet Glendie has brought forth a child of which James Butter acknowledges himself to be the father they did and hereby do find the said parties married persons.

And yet, did some couples feel there was something missing? John Rankine, weaver in Paisley, and Elizabeth McLean in Govan told the latter session in July 1768 that a year earlier they had 'come under Vows & engagements of Marriage to one another and that either that night or within a few days thereafter the Marriage was consummated.' They both looked 'upon themselves as really married to one another tho they are sensible they have transgressed the good order of the Church and desire that their Marriage may still be Celebrated in the usual manner'. The session took some time to deliberate over this matter but in the end agreed that 'upon his producing a Testimonial from Paisley that he is a single person they will appoint the Proclamation of Banns to be Expedite'. There were always going to be some individuals who did not feel truly married without a church wedding, and in fact the nineteenth century saw the fashion for irregular marriage in Scotland largely die out. In our period, however, it made church discipline in the Scottish cities almost impossible to sustain.

Notes

Edinburgh, Canongate and Leith kirk session registers are in the Scottish Record Office; the only exception is Edinburgh New Kirk which for the year 1706 is in Edinburgh University Library and for several other years in Edinburgh City Archive. Aberdeen St Nicholas registers are in Aberdeen City Archive; Old Machar registers are in the parish church, with access via Aberdeen University – microfilms of both sessions' records are in the Scottish Record Office. Glasgow Barony and Govan session registers are in Glasgow City Archive, and have not been microfilmed. Dundee registers are in Dundee City Archive, with microfilms in Edinburgh. We have not given references for each citation but always state the month and year, making it possible for anyone to find a particular case.

1. We wrote a paper on this subject, based on the first portion of our research, entitled 'Clandestine Marriage in the Scottish Cities 1660–1780', which appeared in *Journal of Social History* (Vol. 26, No. 4, Summer 1993).
2. We discussed the subject of regular marriage in some depth in our *Girls in Trouble: Sexuality and Social Control in Rural Scotland 1660–1780* (Edinburgh, 1998), Chapter 3. In Chapter 4 we discussed irregular marriage in the context of our rural parishes.
3. Canon law applied in England as well as in Scotland, and Lawrence Stone discusses this in *Road to Divorce England 1530–1987* (Oxford, 1992), pp. 52–8.
4. *Acts of the Parliaments of Scotland* VII 231 (1661) and X 149b (1698). This information was summarised in Dundee kirk session register in March 1753. At that time – when the English were passing legislation to put a stop to the practice south of the Border – the General Assembly was exerting pressure and requested that an abstract of the laws prohibiting irregular marriage be intimated to every congregation, 'that non may pretend Ignorance'.

8: The Rise and Rise of Irregular Marriage

5 *The Register of the Privy Council of Scotland* V (1676–8), pp. 398–400.
6 Couples who could prove they were 'strangers in this place at the time of their Marriage and were Entirely Ignorant of the Celebrator's Excommunication' were let off.
7 His imprisonment is recorded in Edinburgh Tolbooth Warding and Liberation Books 29 August 1738. SRO.HH110/18. The petition and presbytery's response are recorded in Edinburgh Presbytery minutes 27 September 1738.
8 In October 1742 Isabel Wilson said to Aberdeen session – which contained very few irregularly married couples, for the distance to Edinburgh was too great and there was no local provision – that she had been married to George Loban 'near North Berwick' by David Strang in 1739. She produced marriage lines, but Loban denied being married to her or signing them. Subsequently the session received a letter from David Strang 'with a peremptory denial that he had married George Loban and Isabel Wilson.' Clearly the session had not encountered a marriage certificate of his before but had heard all about him, for it decided that it could pay no regard to Strang's letter, 'he being an infamous person and the session not acquainted with his hand'.
9 Hew Scott, *Fasti Ecclesiae Scotticanae* VI (Edinburgh 1926), p. 122.
10 St Cuthbert's session register August 1754.
11 Edinburgh Tolbooth Warding and Liberation Books 19 June 1758. SRO.HH110/25. He was imprisoned in the Tolbooth on that date and liberated in June 1759.
12 In May 1759 Elizabeth Lees came before South Leith session objecting to the proclamation of banns between William Campbel and another woman, on the grounds that she had been married to him 14 years earlier, and also alleging that Mr Dunning, acting in concert with the session clerk of South Leith, had attempted to bribe her into renouncing all claim to Campbel. Mr Dunning insisted that she 'had quite misapprehended what he spoke to her', and the Leith clerk also denied the charge, but the evidence against them was strong.
13 Mr Lundie thought that 'if the Kirksession of Dundee or any other would complain to the [General] Assembly against the Session Clerk of Edinburgh for his irregular proceedings with regard to Marriage they might find out some ways or means for putting a stop to his irregularity in time coming.'
14 John R. Gillis, *For Better, for Worse: British Marriages, 1600 to the Present* (Oxford, 1985). Irregular marriages virtually ceased in England after Hardwicke's Marriage Act of 1753. There were constant complaints by the English legal establishment over the next two centuries over Scotland's continuing to allow such marriages.
15 We used James Scott Marshall, *Calendar of Irregular Marriages in the South Leith Kirk Session Records 1693–1818* (Edinburgh, 1968), for our irregular marriage figures for this parish. Rosalind Mitchison, reviewing the book for *Scottish Historical Review*, Vol. 49 (1970) counted the number in the marriage register for that period.
16 Lawrence Stone commented, 'One gets the strong impression that the number of bigamists in early modern England must have been quite large.' *Road to Divorce*, p. 142. We get the same strong impression for early modern Scotland.
17 Leah Leneman, *Alienated Affections: The Scottish Experience of Divorce and Separation 1684–1830* (Edinburgh, 1998).
18 In the early years of the Reformation – the 1560s – when no single court was recognised as having consistorial jurisdiction – kirk sessions granted divorces. J.R. Hardy, 'The attitudes of Church and State in Scotland to Sex and Marriage, 1560–1707' (unpublished M.Phil. thesis, Edinburgh University, 1978).
19 Shaw initially refused to submit to discipline on the grounds that his fornication with Margaret Baillie had occurred in England, not Scotland, but he soon gave in.
20 In July 1735 Mary Nicol and Thomas Graham, a soldier, were cited by North Leith session for 'cohabiting as man and wife under a pretence of being married'. They claimed to have been married by David Strang in February but had no certificate to show. 'The session considering that there are more Instances of the like case in this parish were of the mind to wait the Regiments Removal from this place which is expected very soon the Event of

Sin in the City

   which will discover their being Married or not'. But in September the session referred the above case, 'and several other women in this parish who cohabite with the soldiers of Middletons Regiment now gone to Berwick under pretence of a sham marriage' to the presbytery.
21 The 'proper judges' were the Edinburgh commissaries, who dealt with every kind of question connected with marriage; however, bringing a case before them involved hiring lawyers which was obviously a great deterrent.
22 Marriage of Agnes Murray and Andrew Garioch, South Leith, Jan/Feb 1702. The session referred the case to the presbytery for advice on whether to sustain the marriage.

Appendix 9

Total irregular marriages in parishes with long runs

Edinburgh St Cuthbert's
1692–1700: 48
1701–10: 64
1711–20: 101
1721–30: 85
1731–40: 106
1741–50: 142
1751–60: 34
(6 years)

Dundee
1731–40: 17
1741–50: 56
1751–60: 28
1761–70: 29
1771–80: 108
1781–90: 85
1791–1800: 45

South Leith
1691–1700: 38
1701–10: 57
1711–20: 133
1721–30: 132
1731–40: 205
1741–50: 269
1751–60: 278
1761–70: 221
1771–80: 122

North Leith
1711–20: 50
1721–30: 74
1731–40: 101
1741–50: 104
1751–60: 99
1761–70: 110
1771–80: 55

Glasgow Barony
1741–50: 35
1751–60: 20
1761–70: 39
1771–80: 76
1781–90: 204

Glasgow Govan
1741–50: 26
1751–60: 17
1761–70: 24
1771–80: 22
1781–90: 24

Appendix 10

Marriage Case History 1: South Leith

29 September 1720:
James Duncan has just arrived in Leith, alleging that he was married about thirty years ago to Elisabeth Baxter, who had subsequently bigamously married John Alexander and had been living with him as his wife in Leith for the past six or seven years. Duncan appears before the session and produces a declaration signed by various inhabitants of Kirkcaldy, that Duncan and Elisabeth Baxter had been regularly married in the church there in January 1691. Duncan 'affirmed that after they had cohabited together as man & wife a space of 18 weeks, then he was oblidged for bread to go abroad to Holland. After 7 years returning he desired her to cohabite with him; which she refused to do; Then he went to Ireland where he stayed upwards of 4 years, And thereafter returned & lived 4 years in Canongate separately from her, And during these last 4 years, she was living in Leith but refused to cohabite with him & he never took any legal course to oblidge her thereto: After which he went abroad again, and hath stayed abroad ever since till now, being about 13 years; During which space of 13 years foresaid, he affirms that he wrote and sent word to her several times and by several persons... Affirms That it is only Zeall against sin that moves him now to commence this process, And Declares That if John Alexander & she were separated, he is resolved to have nothing to do with her, & will never own nor cohabit with her as his wife; because she is of an intollerable Temper.'

6 October:
Elisabeth Baxter and John Alexander appear. She admits that she was married to James Duncan about thirty years ago but denies that she ever cohabited with him as his wife, 'or that ever she bedded with him, except the first night after their Marriage'. After he returned from abroad the first time she had heard he was in Leith but never saw him. She adds that 'she thought she had good information from several hands... that the said James Duncan was dead before she was married to John Alexander: Likeways she affirmed that the said James Duncan wrote to her within this last quarter of an year, desiring some money from her & he should never trouble her again.' Duncan still insists that they cohabited for 18 weeks. 'He affirmed further that she did see him in Leith, but slighted him, when she saw him', and that 'during the time of his being abroad, he sent home some money & an apron to the said Elisabeth Baxter, but owned that he understood that she would not receive them, & therefore they came to his sister's hands.' Furthermore, he declares that Elisabeth's brother, hearing of the courtship between his sister and John Alexander 'did make search for the said James Duncan at London, & found him... & promised to write to

his sister, shewing her that the said Duncan her Husband was then alive'. John Alexander denies this, saying that 'John Baxter wrote to him about half an year or thereby after his Marriage with the said Elisabeth his sister & wished him joy of his Marriage, & sent him some Tokens or complements, such as Half a Guinea... & a cain staff'. He also says that Elisabeth had assured him that she had good information that her former husband was dead. The session refer the case to the presbytery and forbid Elisabeth Baxter and John Alexander to cohabit in the meantime.

17 November:
The presbytery recommends that the session should write to Kirkcaldy session to get evidence of Duncan's cohabitation with Elisabeth Baxter, and that Duncan should produce evidence of his offering to adhere to Elisabeth when he was last in Scotland. Some witnesses appear but shed no light on the subject.

26 January 1721:
It has now been proved that James Duncan and Elisabeth Baxter 'were publicly married in Kirkcaldy & that they did cohabite some few weeks, but not months'. It is also proven that he stayed in Canongate about 17 years ago but there was no proof 'that he offered to adhere to her, nor her refusing it, nor that she knew of his being alive'. The presbytery 'did find that this process was raised & pursued at the Instance of the said James Duncan only to infer Scandall against the Defenders for Marrying & Cohabiting together, the pursuer being alive, but that he did not pursue for adherence, but declared he would not adhere to her, though the Marriage with John Alexander were declared Null, And that is now about 30 years since he had deserted her, And that he could not make it appear, that in all that time he had ever notified to her his being alive, till about the time of commencing this process or that he desired her to adhere to him, And that he did not pretend any necessary impediment to his adherence, or why he had not notified to her his being Alive, And also Find That she asserted That it was not till after she had heard probable accounts of his death, that she married John Alexander. And Farder They find that the said Defenders Marriage was solemnized according to order after due proclamation of Banns in the parish church where they lived, & that about 23 years after the pursuers desertion. UPON all which it appeared to the Presbytrie that there was no sufficient ground to censure the Defenders for their Marriage or Cohabitation after it, nor to continue them any longer under the prohibition of cohabiting they had been laid under at commencing this process'. As it was clear that Duncan had wilfully deserted his wife thirty years ago and persisted in it, the presbytery judged the first marriage dissolved and that the process should be dropped.

So in this rare case the presbytery actually allowed what was technically a bigamous marriage.

Appendix 11

Marriage Case History 2: South Leith

10 November 1726:
Jasper Cochran and Mary Pollock, who had gone away together last March, returned to the parish a few days earlier. They confess they were irregularly married and produce a certificate. They also confess being guilty of antenuptial fornication. 'He being asked how he came to marry another woman when he had a wife living in the place, with whom he has lived these ten or eleven years. And she being asked how she came to marry a man whom she knew to have a wife alive. He affirmed that altho he lived & cohabited with that woman Janet Ogilvie, yet he was never married with her And the said Mary Pollock said, she knew that he was not married with her.' The session forbid them to cohabit 'untill the process be brought to an Issue'.

1 December:
Janet Ogilvie declares she was married to Jasper Cochran eleven years ago, 'but the said Jasper took away & destroyed the Marriage Lines the Saturday before he went off with Mary Pollock'. Jasper denies the marriage, 'but owned he had lived with & owned her for his wife but was never married, or if it was so, he knew nothing of it, being then so indisposed in health, that he was not able to stand alone, but said, it might be, in that condition, they might cause him to anything; owned when the Ministers came about in the course of visiting families and when the names of families were taken up for examination he gave up his name as husband to the said Janet Ogilvie, & payed the house rent & provided for the family & acted as master thereof but did all that to prevent his being brought to shame, which now he is willing to undergo'. Janet Ogilvie says she can produce witnesses to their marriage.

23 December:
The presbytery advises that the first marriage having been proven before the session, and Janet Ogilvie claiming Jasper as her husband and being willing to adhere to him, Cochran and Mary Pollock are to be forbidden to cohabit.

9 March 1727:
There have been reports of Cochran and Pollock cohabiting. One of the elders went to her house at 4 o'clock in the morning with a constable and an officer and found them both there 'in their shirts' and only one bed in the house. 'Whereupon he caused secure the said Jasper & put him in prison, for cohabiting with the woman after being Discharged both by Session & Presbytrie And that the woman said she would follow him, go where he would.' They confess cohabitation and he is returned to prison and referred to he civil magistrates 'for Execution of the Law'.

Appendix 11

23 March:
She submits herself to discipline and is rebuked 'for her Marrying & living in Adultery with the said Jasper another wifes husband'.

31 August:
The kirk treasurer advises the session he had heard that Jasper Cochran had returned from Holland and was again cohabiting with Mary Pollock. The treasurer had called two constables and two officers 'and went to the house and found him there, holding the child with his clothes loose, ready as appeared to go to bed, Whereupon they put both the said Jasper and Mary in prison.' The moderator told the session that he had visiting Cochran in prison, '& after dealing with him, he confessed that he was Married to Janet Ogilvie in the year of the Rebellion 1715 in some place at the head of the Canongate.' He and Mary appear before the session and they both 'judicially confessed that they have cohabited together since they were Discharged both by Session & Presbytery, but this day, in presence of the Session promised never to cohabit or converse together in time coming.' In view of their past conduct they were returned to prison and referred to the magistrates 'for Execution of the Law'.

This is an example of the full pressure of Church and State being brought to bear on a bigamous couple. In this case there was no doubt of the first marriage, and the first wife wanted her husband back.

Appendix 12

Marriage Case History 3: Edinburgh Canongate

20 August 1745:
It is reported that Agnes Weatherston is married to James Purdie, but Jean Gabriel judicially declares that she was married to Purdie in 1738 by David Strange. He had then been absent from her for five years but returned in July 1744, as a result of which she bore a child in March. She says that 'he broke open her Chest and took out her Marriage Lines and the Letters which he had wrote to her saying that he would leave her Nothing to prove that she was his married Wife.' Agnes Weatherston produces her certificate of marriage with Purdie, saying she knew nothing of a former marriage. She is forbidden to cohabit with him.

3 September:
James Purdie admits cohabiting with Jean Gabriel but denies having been married to her. Witnesses are called.

19 October:
Jean says that since the last meeting of session Purdie 'had twice proffered her money before Witnesses to disclaim her Marriage with him and to desist in the Process before the Session'. More witnesses are called, but Purdie still denies any marriage. He says he offered her two or three shillings 'not to trouble him any more as to The Expences of the child which he owns she bore to him'.

15 February 1746:
Purdie petitions the session, saying that none of the witnesses had proven he was ever married to Jean Gabriel and that she had 'within this month or thereby intermarried with a soldier'.

16 March:
The presbytery finds the marriage between James Purdie and Jean Gabriel proven and that he is therefore guilty of bigamy and adultery and of obtaining a false declaration from Jean Gabriel in which she asserted she was never married to him.

22 April:
Agnes Weatherston declares that she would continue to cohabit with James Purdie and 'would own him as her Husband as long as she lived.' The case is referred back to presbytery.

Appendix 12

10 June:
James Purdie has been laid under the sentence of lesser excommunication. Agnes Weatherston was again prohibited by the presbytery to cohabit with him, but appearing before the session she again asserts that she will cohabit with him as long as she lives. She is referred again to the presbytery.

2 July:
She is laid under the sentence of lesser excommunication but appeals to the synod. Jean Gabriel is now dead. The procurator for the Church is asked whether Purdie could marry Agnes Weatherston, 'with whom he had illegally cohabited dureing the Lifetime of his said first Wife' and declares 'that the said Second Marriage subsists, in the Event of the first being dissolved by death.' As the case is before the synod, the presbytery proceeds no further.

This is an example of the type of case kirk sessions and presbyteries found themselves involved in, and of the difficulty they had in asserting control.

Appendix 13

Marriage Case History 4: Edinburgh Trinity College

Elizabeth Watson is delated for fornication on 22 September 1717. She appears before the session on 12 December and 'Judicially acknowledged That about the first of August last she brought forth a child and that the same was begot with her by John Hamilton Merchant who for present is abroad at the West Indies following his employment But declared that she was married to the said John on the Twenty Eighth of October 1716 in Sir Thomas Wallace his house she being then his servant And being asked if she could produce any Documents for instructing her Marriage could not produce any yea Declared that she knows not so much as the Ministers name that married them and being thereafter asked if she could condescend on the Witnesses names that were present at their Marriage Answered that there were two men present whose names she does not know and one woman called Janet Campbell a widow who then lived near the gates of the said Sir Thomas house And furder Declared that none of the people of that place knew of her Marriage except these two men and that woman And being furder asked how long she was acquainted with the said John Hamilton before their Marriage Answered That she was acquainted with him about a Quarter of a year and that he came from Ireland and being further asked the skippers name of the ship the said John went aboard of Answered that she could not tell but that he went aboard the first of September was a year The Session considering the Lame account she gives in this matter and that they have reason to suspect her Ingenuity [i.e. ingenuousness] They agreed to delay the said Elizabeth till the month of April next to instruct her Marriage'.

17 April 1718:
She is asked for a document proving her marriage but is unable to provide one. The case is referred to the presbytery.

25 June 1719:
The presbytery advises that if she cannot prove her marriage she must satisfy for fornication, and if she cannot prove that the father of her child is a single man, then she must appear as an adulteress.

3 December:
James Cassie appears and declares that he is married to her and the father of her child. Asked 'the time when they were married and by whome and if he had the testificate of their marriage to produce Answered that they were married about Three years agoe by one Mr James Broun in Newton Castle in Sir Thomas Wallace his house near Ayr and declared that he had got a testificate of their Marriage from the

said Mr James but that he had lost it when he went to Sea And being furder asked who were the Witnesses that were present att their Marriage Answered that one John Robertson mariner and Janet Campbell who lives in the West Countrie were both present and did see them married… And the said James being furder asked how long he had cohabite with the said Elizabeth after they were married Answered that he stayed with her about two or three days and then went to Sea being bound for the West Indies and was eighteen months upon that Voyage and declared that he wrote severall letters to the said Elizabeth when he was abroad and furder declared that he was acquainted with her from her infancy and that they were for some time both serving in My Lord Kellies family in Fyffe And being furder asked if he went formerly under the name of John Hamilton Answered that he did indeed go under that name for some Reason known to himself'. The session found that 'there is yet ground to suspect that the abovewritten Account… is neither genuine or so satisfieing as a Case of this nature would require' and referred the case to presbytery.

18 February 1720:
The presbytery had them sign a declaration owning themselves married persons.

One can see from the above why Edinburgh kirk sessions should have become increasingly reluctant to involve themselves in establishing whether pregnant women who claimed to be married were genuinely so.

Appendix 14

Marriage Case History 5: Glasgow Govan

On 22 December 1776 Mary Robertson confesses being with child to William Shiells. He acknowledges being father and also 'that he had promised to marry her and likewise declared that after the report spread abroad that she was with Child he came to her fathers house and desired him to go along and give up their names for Proclamation. That her father at that time refused to go along with him and therefore as her father had refused to go along with him he now had changed his Mind and would not perform his promise at least he would not do it for some time.'

29 December:
Mary 'alledges that he read over to her two Verses in Ruth Ch:1 & v: 16 & 17 and afterwards caused her to read them too and afterwards declared that when this was done that he and she were as really married as any Minister could do it and this was done before he was guilty with her and she believing that this was a real Marriage consented to his desire. He believes that he read these verses mentioned above but does not remember whither or not he called it a real Marriage.

'The Parties being removed the session entered into a solemn deliberation about this unusual affair and holding the parties as being in reality Husband & Wife although without the legal form, they could not admit them to be rebuked before the Congregation as having been guilty of Fornication.

'Then the Parties were called in and this Resolution of the sessions being communicated to them the Moderator earnestly advised William Shiells to acknowledge the Marriage before the session immediately, Upon which he craved a Week to deliberate upon it, which the session agreed to.'

26 January:
'She continues to affirm that before she was got with Child he promised most solemnly to marry her having courted her for that purpose for the space of a twelve Month. He offered a Paper to the session which he was desired to read himself. Its contents were that he was the father of the Child; That he would appear before the Congregation to be rebuked and refused he had promised to marry her and was instantly running off.' The Moderator told him that 'the session were now to deliberate on what sentence should be given in this affair, although he was inticated to stay he ran off declared that he was indifferent what sentence was past.'

2 February:
'in regard it is well known in the Neighbourhood that William Shiells had for a long time courted Mary Robertson which he acknowledges. Acknowledges also he had

Appendix 14

promised to marry her before she consented to be got with Child by him, That he read over the Verses in Ruth Cha:1 16 17 causing her also to read them over, that he declared to her he does not deny that they two were as really married as any Minister could have married them... That after the scandal broke out he offered to give in his Name to the Clerk for proclamation of Banns with her, And considering that when he was solemnly exhorted to acknowledge the Marriage & fulfil his promise publickly he craved only the space of one Week to deliberate on that point. The session think it is clear that William Shiells promised to marry Mary Robertson and that there was a sort of irregular Marriage between William Shiells & Mary Robertson before she was got with Child by him. And therefore the session cannot admit them to undergo Discipline as for Fornication But rather think it expedient that William Shiells be inhibited from marrying any other Woman which may prevent a new Instance of Bigamy if the proper Court shall find that he is already married to Mary Robertson.' The case is referred to the presbytery.

Presbytery minutes 5 March 1777:
Shiells is asked 'Whether he looked upon himself to be under engagements to Mary Robertson as his wife and whether he was willing to adhere to her as such? To both of which he answered in the negative. Parties being removed and the reference read and considered The Presbytery Find no sufficient evidence brought before them of a marriage betwixt the parties. They therefore agree that Mary Robertson should be dismissed after being rebuked by the Moderator and remitt William Shiells to undergo discipline before the Session of Govan'. Shiells was rebuked by the Moderator of the presbytery 'for his prophaness and prevarication'.

In this case the session were in line with a legal definition of marriage in Scotland, which in general the Church – as here represented by Glasgow Presbytery – did not accept.

Appendix 15

Marriage Case History 6: Dundee

2 December 1789:
'Compeared James Finlay of his own accord and informed the session that he having some time ago exchanged Lines with one Catherine Nicoll in promise of a Marriage before two Witnesses viz James Downie & Donald Sime – that he & said Catherine Nicoll some time afterwards having changed their Sentiments with regard to marrying one another they mutually agreed to destroy said Lines which was accordingly done – on account of which he had been kept back from partaking of the Lords Supper & therefore desired that the Session would take the same under Consideration in order that he may be restored to Church Privileges – The Consideration of which was deferred till said Catherine Nicoll & the two Witnesses shall be summoned'.

16 December:
Catherine does not appear but it is reported that 'she was of the same mind with James Finlay viz in declaring that she neither was married to James Finlay nor would she marry him altho he were willing'. James Downie acknowledges seeing the lines, and 'being asked if they acknowledged one another as Man & Wife in said Lines or promised to marry together replied that they were only a promise of Marriage & that as far as he could remember they bore that James Finlay was to marry Catherine Nicoll when convenient for them both'. Donald Sime says that he saw the lines four months earlier and that in them they promised 'to marry one another against Martinmas next & that they did not acknowledge themselves to be married at that time. The Session... were of Opinion that whereas both these Witnesses agreed that the Lines which James Finlay & Catherine Nicoll had exchanged together were only a promise of Marriage & each party having retracted & declared their unwillingness to fulfil their Engagement, there could be no marriage found to subsist betwixt them.'

6 April 1790:
Catherine Nicoll appears with another man, George Malcomb, and they declare that they have been irregularly married. The session is at the same time 'informed that altho they formerly found Catherine Nicoll to be an unmarried Woman according to the Evidence that was then brought before them yet there was reason to suspect that she was really married to James Finlay & was not at liberty to marry any other person while he is alive'. Catherine is asked 'if she thought herself to be at liberty to marry any other man than James Finlay replied that she thought she was free enough when he told her several times he would have nothing to do with her – Being asked

Appendix 15

again & again if she looked upon herself as married to James Finlay when they exchanged Lines together she gave always an evasive Answer. Being asked if she ever lived or cohabited with James Finlay as her Husband she was silent'.

5 May:
Catherine appears and so does James Finlay. She 'declared that she was married to James Finlay about Ten or Eleven Months ago – that as her Father was very much against the Marriage the Lines which they exchanged & which were signed by each party were afterwards destroyed & James Finlay then told her that she might marry whom she pleased so that some time after she in a rage went away with one George Malcomb with a pretence to be married but were not Married – that when they came back James Finlay said where is my Wife going to stay now – which was heard by John Myles & Mungo Allan'. James Downie now declares that to the best of his recollection the content of the lines was: 'I James Finlay lawful son to – Finlay do declare before God & these Witnesses that I take you Catherine Nicoll lawful Daughter of Alexander Nicoll in Hawkhill to be my lawful wedded Wife for better & for worse till God shall separate us by Death or Words to that purpose – he further declared that Catherine Nicoll came to him afterwards to discourse him about said Marriage & refused her being married to James Finlay that he the declarant then told her that if she should marry another man she would be guilty of perjury & that God would deal with her as with one who had broke wedlock... He at the same time declared that he was sorry that he himself had been so far biased by Advice as not to declare all that he knew concerning said Marriage when he was last examined by the Session'. Catherine's brother-in-law also saw the lines and declares likewise. He says that when her parents 'got word of the Marriage they were excessive angry & nothing would satisfy her father but to have these Lines destroyed & the Marriage disannulled & he, the declarant, knew that Catherine Nicoll had no peace nor rest with her Father till she went away with George Malcomb in order to be married and when they returned her father said to the Declarant You was speaking of having a Room taken for her formerly but she behoved to have it now in order that Malcomb & her may be beded – that the declarant was against, however the next Word he heard was that they were beded on Monday Night & came to the Session thereafter in order to have their Marriage confirmed & after they had stayed together for some Days she came to the Declarant & told him that she was repenting of what she had done & would stay no longer with George Malcomb – Upon which he went to her Father to treat with him to take her home again but this her Father would not hear of neither would he have anything to do with her... he the declarant did then take her into his own House in order to keep her from falling into bad Company she having no place to go to. He farther added that he always looked upon the Marriage betwixt James Finlay & Catherine Nicoll as a positive & real Marriage. Catherine Nicoll being farther interrogate with regard to her Marriage continued to declare that she was not married to George Malcomb but that by the advice of her Father... they were beded & lived together nine or 10 Days She also declared that after her Marriage with James Finlay they did cohabit together as Man and Wife altho they did not take up house.' The session finds them 'to be two married persons & that neither of them could marry any other without a legal Divorce & that Catherine Nicoll by her cohabitation with George Malcomb had been guilty of Adultery'.

Sin in the City

19 May:
Catherine's father appears and declares that 'he was against her marrying James Finlay but did not know that she was married to him when she went away [with] another he not having seen the Lines which Finlay & her had exchanged. To which his Daughter answered that he did know that she & James Finlay were married & notwithstanding she could have no peace till she went away with Malcomb in order to be married but was not.' The session decides that as her father 'had acted in so unchristian like manner with regard to his Daughter in his not only advising but in a manner forcing her to commit Adultery he ought to be laid aside from church privileges for some time'.

22 December:
The session decide that as Malcomb 'firmly believed that Catherine Nicoll was an unmarried Woman when he went away with her to be married were of Opinion that he had been guilty of no scandal except a clandestine Marriage… The Session at the same time considering that these clandestine Marriages were often productive of bad Consequences were of Opinion that a Narrative of this affair should be read from the pulpits in order to deter others from such a practice'.

21 October 1791:
Catherine is seven months pregnant in 'adultery' to another man.

12 December 1792:
James Finlay produces 'an Interlocutor obtained by him before the Commissary Court at Edinburgh silencing Catherine Nicoll from calling herself the Wife of said James Finlay – he desired therefore that the Kirk session would find him to be an unmarried man.' Consideration of this is deferred.

The 'bad consequences' of such informal modes of marriage are all too evident in this case.

Conclusion

This book has attempted to record one of the many aspects of life which underwent great change in early modern Scotland. In this period the country's economy, both rural and urban, was transformed, and the bonds holding society together were drastically changed. For the most part they became weaker, but they extended to link people over great distances. The century and a quarter covered by our study saw the closer association of the upper classes of Scotland and England, the agricultural revolution, the development of new areas of trade and new industries, the impact of Enlightenment thought, and the growth of Protestant dissent. Less obvious, and of great relevance to our study, was the acceptance of individualism. Morality ceased to be an area in which the State felt it necessary to intervene, and the Church became less sure of its role. Voluntarism was accepted in religious adherence and manifested itself in the popular attitude to marriage.

Social disapproval of the behaviour of sinners remained an important feature of society, but the Church of Scotland was ceasing to have the accepted authority for their discipline. Sin did not become a neutral matter, let alone an accepted area of activity, but except in the case of professional prostitutes it was coming to be no longer an area for public action. The system of discipline laid down by the Church in the seventeenth century had lost much of its public support, though the Church still retained its authority in matters of dogma. (Dissent did not for the most part mean doctrinal disagreement.)

The change in attitude is a sign of the weakening of the Church as a social organisation, in particular of the loss of effective authority at the level of the urban parish. In some matters what the Church had in the past regarded as its peculiar area of authority had become matters of lay concern and of action by law bodies, for instance town councils or sheriff courts. The Church could no longer expect the sheriff to reinforce its sentence of excommunication, and at the level of ordinary affairs this withdrawal of spiritual privileges left sinners free to join other communions, or to abstain from any form of public worship. In the nineteenth century the Church was to be pushed out of many of its area of social control; it was to see education and poor relief secularised. This trend was already under way in 1780.

But the cities themselves were also losing authority. The tight communities in which everyone knew everybody of note had disappeared. Power was still vested in very few hands but the support of men in lower positions had weakened. No longer could a city close its gates to would-be incomers.

Our particular concern, sexual activity outwith marriage, was coming to be seen as a matter of private, not public, concern. The system of public penance was thought by some to be brutal and undesirable. As religion had become a private matter, so had morality. Indeed, the instances of couples devising their own forms of marriage

Sin in the City

ceremony shows the strength of the desire for private decision making.

Not only do we have to record changes of opinion. Although the old system of discipline continued to function in some rural parishes, it was becoming clear that it could no longer be worked over the country as a whole. There were too many weak spots in the communication network for all sinners to be traced. The sharp fall in the proportion of sinners undergoing discipline in all urban parishes at some point in the eighteenth century is a sign not of effective reformation of behaviour but of inability on the part of the Church courts to keep up with what was going on. Discipline, abandoned early for offences other than sexual, was being dropped in sexual matters because it was impossible to make it comprehensive.

But sexual irregularity did not at the same time become approved behaviour. The self-consciously virtuous continued to disapprove of much of what was going on, but this disapproval had to be expressed in private and personal ways, not with authority.

Index

Aberdeen (New, St Nicholas), 6, 7–8, 12, 13, 14, 15, 17, 21, 24, 30, 31, 34, 35–6, 47–8, 50, 51–4, 56, 62, 65, 70, 74–5, 77–8, 81, 82, 83, 85, 88, 89–90, 92, 93, 94, 95, 100, 101, 104, 105, 107, 108, 112, 116–7, 120–1
   Justice Court, 22–5, 32–3, 70, 75, 81, 82, 83, 84, 85, 88, 89–90, 92, 93, 94, 95, 100, 101, 104, 105, 107, 108, 112, 116–17, 120–1
   presbytery, 47–8, 61, 89, 94
   session clerk, 95–6
Aberdeen, Old (Old Machar), 8, 12, 14, 15, 17, 31, 40, 57, 60, 62, 71, 76, 77–8, 79, 81, 84–5, 94, 95, 98, 100, 103, 110, 111
Aberdeenshire, 75, 77
abortifacients, 54–6, 63
admission levels, 74, 95
agricultural change, 16
Alloa, 87
America, 9
appearances, 20, 92–3
apprentices, 9, 10–11, 98
Argyll, 9
Arnot, H., 21
Ayrshire, 9

Banff, 83
banishment, 30–1, 56
baptism, failure to register, 69
   withholding of, 31
bigamy, 75, 134–5, 146–7, 148–9
Bo'ness, 9
Brechin, 82
bridal pregnancy, 63–5, 71, 77
   in Fife, 72
burgh councils, 21

Calvinism, 2, 4
caution (i.e. surety), 31, 50
child abandonment, 56–8, 62
child support, 86, 104, 107
Church, Episcopal, 13, 41, 43, 86
Church of England, 85
Church of Scotland, 1, 3, 4–5, 7, 13, 15, 16, 17, 31–2, 36, 41, 82

Clark, 20
Cleland, James, 9
cohabitation, 79
consumerism, 14
cottars, 11, 16
craftsmen, 6, 9, 10, 13

Dalmarnock, 101–2
Davies, D., 20, 26, 46
deacons, 19–20, 95
Desbrisay, C.R., 19, 21, 23, 24, 75, 84
dissent, 16, 17, 36, 49, 72, 84–6; *see also* Church, Episcopal, Original Secession, Relief Church
divorce, 5, 133–5
drunkenness, 41, 47, 49
Dundee, 6, 7, 8, 12, 13, 15, 16, 20, 23, 24, 27–8, 31, 36,42, 43, 44, 48, 50–4, 55–6, 57–8, 59, 51–3, 64, 65, 72, 74, 76, 77, 79, 81, 82, 84, 86, 89, 92, 95, 99–100, 102, 104, 105–6, 108, 109, 111, 133–4, 136, 141–2, 145, 156–8
   irregular marriage in, 72, 131, 132
Dunfermline, 5

Edinburgh, 6, 7, 9–11, 14, 15, 17, 20–2, 25–6, 57, 95
   burgh court, 28–9
   correction house, 22, 28
   general session, 20
   Justice of the Peace Court, 29, 46
   Leith, 6, 7, 8, 11, 14, 22, 40, 59
   Portsburgh, 22
   presbytery, 129–30, 131, 141, 148–9, 150–1
   presbytery committee for difficult cases, 89, 90, 97, 98, 103, 107
   university, 14
Edinburgh parishes:
   Canongate, 6, 10–11, 12, 22, 23, 28, 30, 31, 43, 47, 70, 81, 99, 130, 150–1
   Greyfriars, 10
   Greyfriars, New, 14, 51, 70, 81, 86, 94
   Greyfriars, Old, 14, 70, 81, 86, 94, 104, 110

Sin in the City

Lady Yester's, 10, 70, 81
New Kirk, 10, 24, 31, 70, 81, 86, 88, 99, 104–5, 113
North Leith, 11, 12, 29, 47, 52, 57, 59–60, 65, 81, 82, 89, 90, 92, 107–8, 129–30, 132, 133–4, 137, 139–40, 141, 145
Old Kirk, 10, 11, 24, 35, 70, 109, 139
St Cuthbert's, or West Kirk, 2, 10, 12, 24, 26, 31–2, 34, 41, 42, 43–5, 50, 51, 54, 55, 58, 60–1, 62, 64–5, 67–8, 71, 76, 77, 81, 90, 95, 98, 99–101, 104, 105, 107, 109, 110, 112–13, 118–19, 124–5, 129, 130, 131, 133, 139, 145
South Leith, 11, 12, 14, 22, 23, 29, 31, 32, 34, 40–1, 42, 43, 46, 51–3, 54, 56–8, 60, 62, 71, 74, 75, 81, 83, 85, 86, 91–2, 93, 99, 194, 107, 122–3, 132, 137, 139–40, 145, 146–7, 148–9
Tolbooth, 10
Trinity College, 10, 23–4, 26, 30, 31, 34, 41, 50, 62, 70, 71, 76, 81, 85, 86, 93–4, 104, 133, 152–3
Tron, 10, 81
elders, 19, 28, 95
Enlightenment, the Scottish, 14, 15
episcopacy, 8
excommunication, 32
   greater, 32, 130, 135
   lesser, 32, 72, 93, 94, 119, 121

failure of discipline system, 77–8
famine of the 1690s, 13
Fife, illegitimacy in, 72
First Book of Discipline, The, 19
first conceptions out of wedlock, 71–2, 75, 76
flight, 83–4
Forgandenny, 50
Forglen, 83
Form of process, 20
fornication, 5, 19, 21–4
Forty Five rebellion, 13, 31, 66
foundlings, 56–7, 62, 66
France, trade with, 9

General Assembly, 4, 12, 19
gentry, 6, 8, 11, 14, 20, 45–6, 78, 86, 87–8
Glasgow, 6, 7, 9, 12, 13, 14, 15, 16, 36, 86
   presbytery, 132–3, 155
   university, 87
Glasgow parishes:
   Barony, 2, 12, 24, 33, 34, 40, 47, 53, 71, 76, 77, 81, 86, 93, 95, 98, 101, 109–10, 112, 132, 133, 134, 138–9, 141, 145
   Gorbals, 14
   Govan, 12, 33–4, 62, 71, 76, 81, 90–1, 93, 95, 99, 102–3, 112, 126–7, 133, 137–8, 142, 145, 154–5
Glenbervie, 83

hearth tax, 8, 9
Houston, R.A., 21–2
humanitarianism, 16, 35

ignorance, 33
illegitimacy, 1–2, 7, 69–76; *see also* 'repeaters'
industrial development, 17
infanticide, 58–9

Jacobitism, 12–13
James VII, 9, 12

Kemnay, 82
Kilmarnock, 71, 80
King's College, 8
kirk sessions, 4, 7, 19, 20–1, 23, 26, 35, 82
   checking policy of, 82
   persistence of, 83–4
   use of postal service, 82–3
kirk session registers, 75, 81
Kirk treasurers, 25–6

landowners, 12, 87; *see also* gentry
lawyers, 6, 9, 10–1, 12, 20, 86–8
Leith, 6, 7, 8, 11, 14, 22, 40, 42, 59; *see also* Edinburgh
Lothians, illegitimacy in, 76, 77
lying, 98–100, 101–6, 108–11, 112–15, 116–17, 118, 120

McCulloch, Aeneas, 30
Mackenzie, W.M., 21
Man, Isle of, 2
Marischal College, 8
marriage, 4–5
   expectations of, 62
   promise of, 62–5, 126
marriage, irregular, 90, 128–42, 148–50, 153, 156–8
   celebrators of, 129–31
   claims of, 71, 72
   motives for, 128, 131–2
   penalties, 128
membership of congregation, 36

162

Index

merchants, 6, 10–1, 13
midwives, 51, 53–4, 57, 64, 65, 67–8, 92, 103, 104, 107, 108, 109, 110, 124–5
  bond of, 67–8
misnaming, 104, 107–9, 112–3, 116, 120, 122–3, 124–5
mistaken identity, 108
Monifieth, 108

Navigation Act, 9
Netherlands, trade with, 8, 9
  wars with, 12

Oath of Purgation, 88, 102–4, 113, 115, 126, 127
Original Secession, 16

Paterson, David (irregular marriage celebrator), 130
Perth, 6, 51
pew renting, 72, 80
physicians, 6, 9
poll tax, 8, 9, 11, 12
Port Glasgow, 9
premarital pregnancy, 5, 20
presbyterianism, 12
presbyteries, 4, 19, 106, 109, 113, 115, 126–7
  appeal to, 121
presumption of guilt, 103–6, 125
Privy Council, 40
prostitutes, 30–1
prostitution, 21
Protestantism, 97

Quakers, 84
Queensferry, 100

rape, 30, 60–1
recalcitrance, 82–4, 86–7, 88–95, 98–115
recalcitrant women, 90–3, 116–17
Reformation, 19
Relief Church, 16
'repeaters', 69, 71, 75, 77–9
reputation, 99–101
Revolution (of 1689), 9, 12, 13

Roman Catholicism, 4
Roman Catholics, 84–5
Royal Burghs, 7
  tax on, 8–9

sackcloth, 92, 111
sailors, 89, 132
St Ninian's, 86
Schilling, Heinz, 32
Scots Magazine, 35
servants, 110–11, 59
service, 5, 11
Session, Court of, 9, 12
Sexuality and Social Control, 1
social control, 7, 70
soldiers, 24, 75, 89–90, 132, 136–7, 144
South Uist, 90
Statistical Account of Scotland, The, 70
Stone, Lawrence, 142
Strang, David, (irregular marriage celebrator), 129–30, 132
surgeons, 9
synods, 4, 19

Tay ports, 8
'testificates' (testimonials), 35, 101
threats, 111–12
Trustees, Board of, 13
Tucker, Thomas, 8

Union, Act of (1707), 13
universities, 15
'unknown man', 109–11
urban growth, 6, 15, 72

venereal disease, 66
voluntarism, 36

weavers, 10
Webster, Alexander, census by, 14, 70
Western Isles, 9
wet nursing, 57
whipping, 56
witchcraft, 42–3
witnessing, of irregular marriages, 140–1